Initiating Therapy in
HEART FAILURE

Iain B Squire

BSc MBChB FRCP MD

Senior Lecturer in Medicine, University of Leicester and
Honorary Consultant Physician, University Hospitals of Leicester

**This independent educational book has
been donated as a service to medicine
by**

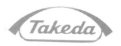

MAGISTER CONSULTING LTD

INITIATING THERAPY IN HEART FAILURE
by IAIN B SQUIRE BSc MBChb FRCP MD

Published in the UK by
Magister Consulting Ltd
The Old Rectory
St. Mary's Road
Stone
Dartford
Kent DA9 9AS

Copyright © 2005 Magister Consulting Ltd
Printed in the UK by Nuffield Press Ltd, Abingdon, Oxon.

ISBN 1 873839 65 0

About the Author

Iain B Squire BSc, MBChB, FRCP, MD
Senior Lecturer in Medicine, University of Leicester and
Honorary Consultant Physician, University Hospitals of Leicester

Iain Squire is Senior Lecturer in Medicine, University of Leicester, and Consultant Physician at University Hospitals of Leicester. He trained in Glasgow and Leicester. His specialist interests are in acute coronary syndromes and CHF. Dr Squire has published extensively in these areas with over 60 original papers and book chapters.

Foreword

With an overall incidence of 1%, rising to 30% in those over 80 years, primary care clinicians have to deal with acute and chronic heart failure on a regular basis. The importance of this condition has been recognised by its inclusion as one of the key therapeutic areas in the new general medical services contract for General Practitioners in the UK.

The greater availability and power of diagnostic and imaging tools, a more sympathetic approach to the frightening connotations to the patient of the term "heart failure" and a variety of useful therapeutic interventions, both pharmacological and physical, have reversed the nihilism and fear associated with this condition for patient and clinician alike.

Rarely can a syndrome have seen such a dramatic change in the pharmacological approach to its management. Not only have traditional therapies been superseded by the introduction of new powerful and effective agents, but there has been a revolution in the use of a therapy class. ß adrenoceptor antagonists were once strictly contraindicated in heart failure. Now it is clear that, if used judiciously, they can be extremely beneficial.

In this book, Dr Iain Squire describes the classification, diagnosis, pathophysiology and treatment of heart failure. The focus is always on the clinical management of the patient and the roles and responsibilities of different disciplines. Where necessary, clinical trial data are presented and referenced; the basic sciences of pathology and pharmacology are used to explain the clinical approach.

Dr Squire's cautious, careful and considered style denotes his active clinical background and a thoughtful approach to a condition that cannot be dealt with lightly. This book will appeal to primary care clinicians, hospital staff and students seeking background and guidance on the contemporary management of heart failure.

John Haughney, 25th September 2005

Contents

CHAPTER ONE

Introduction

Background

Heart failure is a common and disabling condition. As a result of improvements in survival after myocardial infarction and, partly as a result of the ageing of the population in industrialised societies, heart failure has increased in prevalence over the last 30 years. As the only manifestation of coronary heart disease to be increasing in incidence, it now constitutes one of the largest components of health care costs in developed countries. The high costs to the health care community are consequent upon the lack of ability for self-care and the frequent hospital admissions that the condition generates.

However, over the same period there has been a revolution in the perception of heart failure by health care professionals. The development of effective treatments has turned heart failure from what was once considered a terminal illness with a bleak prognosis into an area of considerable therapeutic interest. Inhibitors of the renin-angiotensin system, the angiotensin-converting-enzyme (ACE) inhibitors and angiotensin receptor blockers (ARB) reduce mortality, improve symptoms and delay the progression of heart failure, as well as modifying the ventricular remodelling process which may lead to heart failure after myocardial infarction.

The beta-blockers once considered as absolutely contraindicated in heart failure have shown clear therapeutic benefits across a wide spectrum of severity of chronic heart failure and in heart failure after acute myocardial infarction (AMI). At the other end of the treatment spectrum, transplantation and other surgical options have evolved. Surgical therapies for heart failure now constitute viable treatment options for some groups of patients.

The use of either temporary or permanent implantable mechanical assist pump devices provides a possible bridge or alternative to transplantation.

Implantable defibrillator devices are being employed to protect against malignant ventricular arrhythmias. Cardiac resynchronisation therapy (CRT) provides profound symptomatic improvement in a proportion of patients and has very recently been shown to improve life expectancy. Finally, poorly functioning, but potentially viable, ventricular myocardium, a condition termed hibernating myocardium, can be restored to better function by surgical revascularisation.

Importantly, the quality of patients' lives can be improved by specialised nursing, dietician and rehabilitation care including substantial improvements in exercise capacity in selected patients by tailored physical training programmes. What was once an area of therapeutic despair is now one of considerable opportunity. Central to the changing management of heart failure has been the development of heart failure specialists at secondary care, primary care and nursing level. This monograph aims to instruct the clinician in modern thinking on the assessment and treatment of heart failure, and how to manage these new treatments within contemporary practice.

Epidemiology

In the United Kingdom, the incidence of heart failure is about 20 to 30 per thousand per year and the overall prevalence of the condition in the population is about one per cent. Heart failure is increasingly common with age, reaching 30 per cent prevalence in those over the age of 80[1]. Increasing longevity in industrialised societies means there are more elderly people; as a result heart failure is an increasingly important personal, and public, health care issue.

Paradoxically, improvements in the management of acute myocardial infarction (AMI) and chronic coronary heart disease have led to more heart failure rather than less: survivors of acute cardiovascular episodes develop heart failure later in life. Moreover, each treatment advance that reduces mortality after AMI and in chronic heart failure actually increases the number of patients with the condition within a health care community at any one time.

Chronic heart failure is characterised by frequent symptomatic relapses, resulting in frequent acute hospital and long-stay residential care admissions. It is estimated to be the single most common reason for admission to hospital in people over the age of 65, and also the most expensive single diagnosis. The rate of re-admission to hospital after discharge is also higher for heart failure than any other condition. In part by virtue of its having many possible aetiologies, and in part due to its being increasingly prevalent with greater age, heart failure is associated with multiple comorbidity, factors which often complicate the management of the condition. For all these reasons, heart failure is of major importance in both health economics and life quality in an ageing society.

Classification

Historically, heart failure was classified by the predominant clinical pattern of the syndrome into 'forward' heart failure where the condition was dominated by the features of low cardiac output and reduced perfusion of vital organs with renal failure, hypotension, and hepatic dysfunction, or 'backward' failure where the clinical presentation was dominated by pulmonary and venous congestion[2]. A similar idea lies behind the terms congestive heart failure and non-congestive heart failure.

With the development of powerful diuretic agents and the use of short-term inotropic or mechanical assist devices, intractable oedema is now very rare, and the most common syndrome is the non-oedematous but still markedly limited patient with symptoms of fatigue and dyspnoea on low levels of physical effort. In such patients, resting clinical signs and even haemodynamic measurements may be remarkably normal despite the severe symptomatic limitation.

Many of the symptoms in these patients are probably produced by an array of extra-cardiac complications that develop (see the pathophysiology section below). This clinical picture has been termed the 'Syndrome of Chronic Heart Failure' [3], which, for simplicity's sake, I will abbreviate as CHF for the rest of the monograph.

Other systems of classifying types of presentation of heart failure are used where helpful to describe the cause or nature of the heart failure more accurately. An acute episode of heart failure producing severe pulmonary oedema and perhaps cardiogenic shock is called acute heart failure, whereas a patient with no signs of acute decompensation but evidence of abnormal left ventricular function and symptomatic limitation is described as suffering from chronic heart failure. Ventricular dysfunction due to left ventricular disease is called left heart failure, when only the right ventricle is affected it is termed right heart failure, and when both ventricles are affected, bi-ventricular failure.

In simple terms, heart failure is a condition where symptoms of exercise intolerance are caused by objective impairment of cardiac function[2]. This is a clinically useful definition which does not depend on specialised investigations or invasive monitoring, but which defines a patient group with similar problems who might benefit from similar therapeutic approaches.

One other classification is likely to be of increasing interest in the future, and that is of the primary abnormalities of the function of the left ventricle. In most cases of heart failure, there is reduction in the force of cardiac contraction, and the left ventricle is enlarged with reduced systolic function. In a smaller number of patients, systolic left ventricular contraction may appear to be within normal limits, but the heart cannot fill adequately without excessively high ventricular filling pressures. These people can have severe symptoms of exercise intolerance and pulmonary congestion and suffer what is described as heart failure with preserved systolic function (sometimes referred to as diastolic as opposed to systolic heart failure).

This situation, especially common in older patient groups, can be recognised accurately only by detailed echo-Doppler studies or invasive monitoring. Clinically this entity is often extremely difficult to identify with certainty. It can, however, be suspected clinically in patients with classical extra-cardiac manifestations of heart failure despite a normal or small-sized heart with preserved systolic function on echocardiography. The patient usually has hypertension or a history thereof. The importance of identifying heart failure with preserved systolic function lies in the fact that the response to treatment, vasodilators in particular, may be different to that of the more common systolic heart failure.

Table 1 lists the major causes of heart failure subdivided by the predominant pathophysiological mechanism.

Table 1: **Major causes of heart failure based on the principal mechanism of cardiac dysfunction**

1. Loss of myocytes	Infarction Idiopathic myocyte necrosis Infective cardiomyopathies, e.g. respiratory viral infection, Chagas' disease, HIV Toxic cardiomyopathies, e.g. alcohol, chemotherapy Infiltrations: sarcoid, amyloid, iron overload
2. Myocyte dysfunction	Some idiopathic or familial cardiomyopathies Chronic ischaemia ('hibernating myocardium') Endocrine disorders, e.g. thyrotoxicosis, hypocalcaemia, acromegaly Hypertrophic cardiomyopathy Restrictive cardiomyopathy
3. Alterations in myocardial interstitium	Senile fibrosis Endomyocardial fibrosis Pathological fibrotic hypertrophy, e.g. hypertension
4. Valvular disorders	Calcific, congenital or rheumatic valve disease Degenerative disease, e.g. myxomatous degeneration of the mitral valve Infective endocarditis Non-infective endocarditis, e.g. secondary to connective tissue diseases
5. Pericardial disorders	Constrictive pericarditi Cardiac tamponade

Aetiologies

Heart failure is a clinical syndrome, not a single diagnosis, and may be the result of any one, or a combination of, pathological processes. In industrialised societies the single most common underlying cause of heart failure is ischaemic heart disease, followed by hypertension, and idiopathic dilated cardiomyopathy[4]. In hospital practice, increasing numbers of patients are seen with heart failure secondary to chemotherapy for malignancy, a sign of improved survival from these cancers. In the third world and the tropics, valvular disease, rheumatic heart disease and nutritional deficiencies constitute more significant causes.

Some geographical areas have specific diseases which may predispose to heart failure, such as Chagas' disease in South America, iron overload in certain populations in southern Africa and nutritional deficiency states in the world's poorest countries. It is important to note that there is also an increasing prevalence of AIDS cardiomyopathy in sub-Saharan Africa, and to a lesser extent in Western countries.

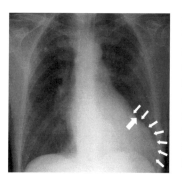

FIGURE 1.1 – **Chest X-Ray from a patient with heart failure secondary to anterior MI several years previously. The patient had occluded left coronary artery with no reversible ischaemia beyond the occlusion; revascularisation was not indicated. The dark arrows outline a left ventricular aneurysm. The lighter arrow indicates an area of calcification within thrombus contained in the aneurysm.**

In practice, it may be difficult to identify with confidence the aetiology of heart failure; indeed, a combination of pathological factors may contribute to heart failure in an individual patient. Many cases of heart failure in a patient with coronary artery disease and a few with dilated heart and globally impaired ventricular function may involve a contribution from previously undetected or poorly treated hypertension, 'burnt-out' by the time of presentation due to the reduction in the force of cardiac contraction.

Diagnosis

Heart failure is both one of the most simple and one of the most elusive of diagnoses. Determining the cause of pulmonary oedema in the patient suffering a massive myocardial infarction is not difficult, but determining the contribution of heart failure to dyspnoea and ankle oedema in an elderly woman with a small heart on chest X-ray can be extremely difficult.

A diagnosis of heart failure depends on the presence of symptoms consistent with this diagnosis (exertional dyspnoea and fatigue in excess of those expected for the patient's age and degree of fitness), combined with some objective evidence of reduction in cardiac function, either systolic or diastolic. For many patients clinical examination and chest radiography may be sufficient, whereas in others echocardiography and possibly even cardiac catheterisation for detailed pressure recording may be required.

Recent years have seen the emergence of the natriuretic peptides as aids to diagnosis in the patient in whom heart failure is suspected. In practice, these peptides are excellent at ruling out heart failure, when the plasma level is within the reference range. However, when raised above this level the positive predictive value is low, particularly in elderly populations. The place of the natriuretic peptides in standard clinical practice remains to be established fully.

Summary

Heart failure is increasingly common, debilitating and lethal. It can be classified into acute or chronic, congestive or non-oedematous, systolic or diastolic and left, right or bi-ventricular. Heart failure may also be usefully classified according to aetiology.

The major causes of heart failure in the developed world are ischaemic heart disease and hypertension. Major treatment advances have occurred in the last decade, the most important of which are the introduction of the inhibitors of the renin-angiotensin system (ACE inhibitors, ARBs, aldosterone antagonists) and beta-blockers. Treatment advances over the last few years now offer the real possibility of symptomatic improvement for what used to be considered a hopeless and untreatable condition.

CHAPTER TWO

Pathophysiology

The heart

In heart failure there are changes in the size, shape, structure and function of the heart, particularly in the left ventricle. In the most common type of heart failure — left ventricular systolic dysfunction — the clinical picture usually includes enlargement of the left ventricular cavity which becomes more spherical. The change in ventricular shape, whilst initially being an adaptive response to ventricular wall stress and thereby myocardial oxygen consumption, can become maladaptive.

Advances in medical imaging have demonstrated how the normal ventricle contracts in a process similar to wringing out a dish-mop. The apex of the heart contracts first with a twisting motion which moves blood into the base of the heart forming a small, more spherical cavity which then pushes the blood as a bolus out into the ascending aorta.

During this process, the mitral valve apparatus is pulled towards the apex of the heart so that, during diastole, the opposite motion produced by active recoil of the ventricle causes the mitral valve apparatus to move over and incorporate a volume of blood from the left atrium. This is an elegant and very energy-efficient process. The failing ventricle loses this organised contractile function, which becomes incoordinate and inefficient. The size of the heart is known to be a marker of prognosis independent of other aspects of severity, and the shape-change is probably also a detrimental feature of advanced heart disease.

The process of ventricular enlargement has received considerable attention recently as this process is thought to contribute to the development of heart failure after a large myocardial infarction in a process termed ventricular 'remodelling' [5, 6]. It is thought that the physical strain on the recently infarcted myocardium causes enlargement of the apparent area of the infarct scar (infarct expansion), a process quite distinct from further infarction (infarct extension).

Later, over weeks to months, the residual healthy myocardium can adapt to altered loading conditions and neurohormonal activation by slipping of cell-to-cell junctions, leading to the remodelled and enlarged ventricle of CHF. The observation that inhibitors of the renin-angiotensin-aldosterone system can delay or prevent this process underlies the exciting developments of their use in the post-infarction period.

The failing heart also shows alterations in cardiac structure at microscopic and ultra-structural levels. The increased wall stress and neurohormonal activation characteristically seen after a large myocardial infarction or in early heart failure can lead to an increase in the collagen content of the ventricular wall. Angiotensin II and, particularly, aldosterone are thought to contribute to this process which, although initially adaptive, eventually leads to possibly irreversible myocardial fibrosis.

This change reduces ventricular wall distensibility and may also adversely affect the diastolic filling process, reducing the efficiency of converting contractile protein cross-bridge formation into ventricular contraction. As a result, these microscopic structural changes can explain worsening of both systolic and diastolic function in the enlarging ventricle of CHF.

There are a number of other changes in the microscopic structure of the failing ventricle with a reduced number of tight junctions between myocytes, slipping of connections between myocytes and an abnormal load per myocyte. All of these alterations affect the mechanical and electrical performance of individual cells and the interactions between cells. These changes are thought to be responsible for some of the electrical instability of the failing heart and likely contribute to the high incidence of apparently random ventricular arrhythmias that characterise CHF.

The circulation

The left ventricle is a pump which generates both pressure and flow. The energy it imparts to the blood during each heartbeat can be measured as the average cardiac power output (flow x mean blood pressure). The healthy heart works within its maximum cardiac power output, the reserve capacity being called upon when increased output is required, e.g. in exercise. The overall reserve cardiac power output is dramatically reduced in severe heart failure and such a reduction is a marker of a poor prognosis[7].

Power output is not easily measured in clinical practice but we can measure the components of cardiac function by measuring blood pressure, cardiac output and intra-cardiac filling pressures. This approach is particularly useful in the management of acute heart failure where the aim of therapy is to correct haemodynamic status. Provided an adequate filling pressure (pre-load, adequate left ventricular end-diastolic pressure or LVEDP) exists, low cardiac output may be treated by positive inotropic agents.

If the LVEDP is elevated this is transmitted to the pulmonary veins leading to eventual extravasation of fluid into the alveoli and pulmonary oedema. Direct measurement of pulmonary venous pressures is impossible but can be estimated from the pulmonary capillary wedge pressure. This is the pressure in a Swan-Ganz catheter tip just before the inflated balloon tip occludes the pulmonary artery lumen and allows the catheter tip pressure to equilibrate with that of the pulmonary venules and the left atrial pressure.

This wedge pressure is particularly useful in managing acute heart failure; too low a wedge pressure will reduce cardiac output and too high a wedge pressure will produce pulmonary oedema. The correct choice of inotropic agents, vasodilators, diuretics and mechanical assist devices can be made only by careful assessment of the central haemodynamic status of which, in the very sick patient, pulmonary artery pressure monitoring by Swan-Ganz catheter is an important component.

Systolic function

Systolic function can be estimated by haemodynamic measurements. Left ventricular systolic dysfunction will show reduced peak rate of pressure rise within the ventricle (positive dP/dt max.) and increased filling pressure (LVEDP). In systolic dysfunction, the failing ventricle utilises its Frank-Starling mechanism reserve and operates at large ventricular volumes with high filling pressures.

Ventriculography (either radiographic or radio-nuclear) or echocardiography can measure end-diastolic and end-systolic volumes and derive the ejection fraction (the fractional emptying of the ventricle).

Left ventricular ejection fraction (LVEF) is a popular and useful way of grading the systolic function. LVEF has the advantage of simplicity and is an important predictor of longevity in heart failure, independent of other measures of severity[8]. Normal ranges for LVEF vary between laboratories and the method of estimation, but above 60 per cent is considered normal, below 40 per cent significantly impaired, and below 20 per cent severe dysfunction.

At the simplest level, LVEF gives an easily recognisable description of the degree of systolic dysfunction in heart failure. However, LVEF correlates only poorly with the degree of symptomatic limitation in patients with the syndrome of CHF. This is also true for haemodynamic measures, reflecting the importance of non-cardiac changes in the genesis of symptoms in this syndrome.

Diastolic dysfunction

Diastole is the period of filling of the ventricle prior to the next heartbeat. Objective measurements of diastolic function are, however, more problematic than for systolic function. Whereas systole occurs rapidly and in one action, diastole is complex, with an initial rapid and active ventricular recoil producing rapid filling of the ventricle, followed by a period of relative stasis as atrial and ventricular pressures equilibrate, then a second period of ventricular filling produced by the effects of atrial contraction.

The presence of atrial fibrillation, A-V block, or even changes in heart rate interfere with these relationships so that no simple, reliable measure exists of the adequacy of diastole. The measures of diastolic function which are used, such as the ratio of early to atrial (E to A) velocities of transmitral blood flow, or the peak rate of ventricular filling on radionuclide ventriculography depend importantly on systolic function, heart rate, and the degree of sympathetic stimulation. The difficulty in identifying and quantifying diastolic dysfunction is illustrated by the very poor correlations which exist among a variety of echocardiographic measures of this entity[9].

Diastolic functional disturbance remains important, however. There are cases of definite clinical heart failure in which the patient has a small heart with normal or even increased left ventricular ejection fraction, and in whom the only demonstrable abnormalities of ventricular mechanics are those related to ventricular relaxation and filling (diastole). This pattern of heart failure is uncommon in ischaemic heart disease but is seen with increasing frequency in older patient groups in whom senile myocardial fibrosis occurs more frequently as the major pathology underlying the heart failure. Another common scenario is the patient with hypertension, LV hypertrophy and perhaps renal impairment.

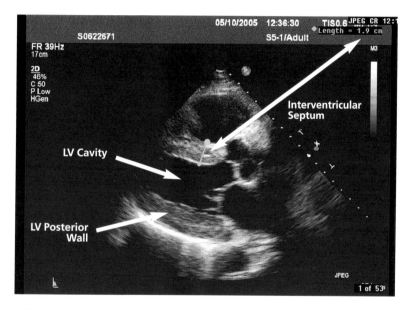

FIGURE 2.1 – *echocardiographic findings in a 63 year old patient with previous CABG, peripheral vascular disease, renal impairment and now presenting with frank heart failure. LV systolic function was preserved. The echocardiogram shows marked LV hypertrophy with almost complete obliteration of the LV cavity during systole. This is a clear example of heart failure with preserved systolic function.*

Other rarer causes include hypertrophic cardiomyopathy and infiltrative conditions such as amyloid heart disease.

Pericardial pathology is a rare cause of heart failure, but one which should not be forgotten. Pericardial constriction and tamponade are treatable conditions which can complicate connective tissue diseases, infections, open heart surgery, tuberculous pericarditis or carcinoma of the lung, or mediastinum. When heart failure is present on a background of one of these underlying conditions, it should lead to physical examination looking for evidence of tell-tale signs: Kussmaul's sign (an increase in central venous pressure with inspiration), and pulsus paradoxus (a reduction in arterial and pulse pressure on inspiration).

In pericardial constriction there is an elevated jugular venous pressure and a rapid x-descent in the jugular venous pulse. A globular heart shadow may be seen on chest X-ray in pericardial tamponade and may be the only investigative feature prior to the most definitive test: echocardiography. Treatment may be life-saving and includes either percutaneous pericardial tap or surgical production of a pericardial window to drain the fluid.

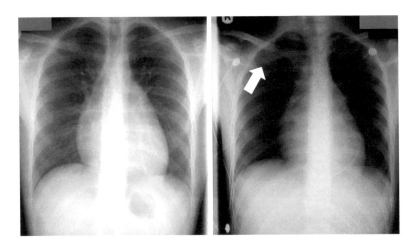

Figure 2.2: **Chest x-ray images before and after insertion of pericardial drain. The image on the left shows cardiomegaly in a patient who presented with typical features of pericardial effusion. In the second image, a pericardial drain is in-situ and there is clear reduction in the size of the cardiac contour. The arrow shows a Ghon focus of TB, the cause of the pericardial effusion in this case.**

Non-cardiac abnormalities
in chronic heart failure

CHF is a multi-system disorder in which modern pharmacological therapy can almost completely correct the oedema and pulmonary congestion and even largely correct the resting haemodynamic abnormalities. However, major symptomatic limitation often remains and to explain this we must turn our attention to pathophysiological processes in other organ systems.

The major symptoms of patients with CHF are dyspnoea on mild to moderate exertion and muscle fatigue. Study after study has shown that the central haemodynamics in these patients cannot explain why these symptoms occur. Hence, we do not know the best way to treat them.

In acute exacerbations with pulmonary oedema, shortness of breath is the major symptom. In the majority of patients with CHF, shortness of breath is not accompanied by pulmonary congestion and it is difficult to explain this common symptom. It is usually proposed that there must be a mis-match between blood flow to, and ventilation of, the lungs, the dyspnoea being produced by excessive dead-space ventilation.

There is little convincing evidence for this, and alternative explanations exist. The signal for dyspnoea may be generated elsewhere in the body, perhaps via a perception of the effort needed for exercise, or by a signal from the exercising muscle or the respiratory muscles, both of which are excessively metabolically stressed during exercise. There is evidence in CHF for excessive and early release of the products of muscular exercise, which include lactic acid, potassium and adenosine. But whether these and other factors can explain this disabling symptom remains uncertain[10].

We understand a little bit more about the genesis of the symptoms of muscle fatigue which afflict patients with CHF. There is a reduction in blood flow to the exercising skeletal muscle in these patients, probably more to do with the loss of muscle in the periphery and excessive vasoconstriction of the muscle vasculature than to acute impairment of the pumping capacity of the heart. Thus attempts to increase the cardiac output acutely with positive inotropic agents do not improve either skeletal muscle blood flow or exercise tolerance. Even cardiac transplantation takes many weeks for this to improve, possibly because of the time taken to correct the peripheral abnormalities which usually generate the fatigue.

There are considerable changes within the skeletal muscle of patients with CHF which may explain these observations[11]. These changes include a considerable loss of muscle mass (cardiac cachexia when severe), an alteration in the structure of the muscle macroscopically and microscopically, and impaired muscular function and metabolism. These changes have been found to explain muscle fatigue far better than parameters of either left ventricular or central haemodynamic function. Thus the periphery may be an important area for both the generation of symptoms in CHF and for potential therapeutic measures to improve these symptoms[12].

It is important to note that deconditioning secondary to inactivity contributes to the progression of muscle weakness and symptoms of fatigue in CHF; exercise rehabilitation can markedly improve exercise capacity.

The vasculature

Microvasculature changes occur in many organ systems and these may contribute to the organ under-perfusion and dysfunction seen in the syndrome of CHF. Endothelial-dependent vasomotor control systems are disordered with a reduction in the natural vasodilator system of endothelial-derived relaxing factor (EDRF) and excessive activity of the vasoconstrictor system, endothelin.

The natriuretic peptide system, powerfully vasodilator, is activated in CHF. Indeed, while the site of production of atrial and B-type natriuretic peptides is the cardiac ventricles, C-type natriuretic peptide (CNP) appears to be produced by the vascular endothelium[13].

Generalised endothelial dysfunction may contribute to renal, hepatic and pulmonary vascular impairment. Specific treatments for endothelial abnormalities have not been described for heart failure but are possibly affected by ACE inhibitors or physical training. There is particular interest in endothelin, both because raised levels are associated with a poor outcome in heart failure, and because of the development of antagonists against the receptors stimulated by endothelin[14]. Disappointingly, clinical trials of endothelin antagonists in the management of CHF have failed to show any therapeutic benefit[15].

The function of even the large conduit arteries is abnormal in CHF. This produces decreased arterial compliance and reduces the efficiency of ventriculo-aortic coupling, leading to further work for the failing left ventricle. The large arterial changes are secondary to sympathetic and possibly local renin-angiotensin system activation within the arterial wall. Again, the natriuretic peptide system may have pathophysiological significance in this regard.

The lungs

The volume, structure, strength and fatiguability of respiratory musculature are abnormal in CHF. Respiratory muscle fatigue which is well recognised in end-stage lung disease is now recognised in CHF. It may be important in generating the sensation of dyspnoea, in limiting exercise tolerance, and in the production of nocturnal episodes of hypoxia in these patients, which some believe may predispose to sympathetic over-activity and ventricular arrhythmias. Indeed, disordered respiratory patterns, particularly during sleep, are associated with adverse outcome in CHF.

Lung structure itself may be chronically abnormal in CHF and, in severe cases, secondary pulmonary hypertension, due to irreversible pulmonary arterial changes, can develop and lead to right ventricular failure. This is much more common in mitral stenosis than in left ventricular failure itself. There is evidence that a diffusion limitation for oxygen can occur within the lungs of patients with CHF but the extent to which this can explain the reduction in exercise capacity in CHF remains very controversial[16].

It is a fact that arterial blood gases are remarkably normal even during exercise in patients with CHF, suggesting that this diffusion limitation is easily compensated and is not of major pathophysiological importance. Hypoxaemia is very rare during exercise in patients with CHF[17] and, where seen, should prompt a search for an alternative explanation such as pulmonary emboli, independent lung disease or the presence of a right to left shunt of blood across the lungs, thereby delivering de-oxygenated blood to the arterial circulation.

Many patients with CHF, even when lifelong non-smokers, can complain of a wheezy sensation which can be very difficult to differentiate from asthmatic bronchospasm. It is believed that bronchial mucosal oedema can lead to a hyper-responsiveness to bronchoconstrictor stimuli, producing the syndrome of cardiac asthma. Where both heart and lung disease co-exist both the patient and the physician know the difficulty in differentiating which component is causing any particular exacerbation of dyspnoea.

On provocation tests there is little evidence for bronchial hyper-reactivity in CHF provided care is taken to control the confounding effects of patients with CHF who have been frequent heavy smokers and hence have another reason for bronchial constriction[18].

Control of breathing

Increased sensitivity of arterial chemoreceptors to hypoxia, and central chemoreceptors in the brain stem to carbon dioxide, are apparent in stable CHF[19]. This may explain both the heightened ventilatory response to exercise of the patient with heart failure (they seem to breathe more than they need to) and could help explain some of their sensation of dyspnoea.

The associated findings that the chemoreceptors are a powerful sympathetic nervous system stimulant and are intimately involved in the generation of Cheyne-Stokes respiratory pattern and central sleep apnoea, may explain some hitherto unexplained observations in heart failure - that of the cause of persistent sympathetic drive, sleep apnoea and Cheyne-Stokes respiration. Treatments that reduce chemosensitivity can increase exercise capacity in heart failure patients, but no clinically practicable treatment has as yet been developed[20].

The pattern of breathing in heart failure is abnormal with a preference for inefficient rapid shallow respiration. There is an increased frequency of central sleep apnoea in heart failure patients and this may contribute to the rate of nocturnal ventricular arrhythmias; hypoxaemia during sleep results in major surges in sympathetic tone to the heart as chemoreceptor drive kicks in after each apnoeic episode. In addition, these episodes may impair sleep quality and adversely affect daytime alertness and quality of life.

Reports of daytime somnolescence should always raise the possibility of nocturnal hypoxaemia. Nocturnal oxygen supplementation may offer several potential advantages to the patient with severe heart failure. Indeed, CPAP (continuous positive airways pressure) is used increasingly in CHF patients with abnormal nocturnal breathing patterns. While a proportion fail to tolerate CPAP, at least as many achieve significant symptomatic improvement with relief of daytime somnolescence, greater alertness and better quality of life.

Skeletal muscle

In CHF there is reduced peak strength and early fatiguability of skeletal muscle[11]. Patients often complain that muscle fatigue is the major limitation to the performance of their daily tasks.

Skeletal muscle metabolism during exercise is also profoundly abnormal whether the heart failure is due to dilated cardiomyopathy or secondary to ischaemic heart disease. There is early depletion of phosphocreatine which contains high energy phosphate bonds and early acidification during exercise. These changes cannot be explained by the acute effects of impaired blood flow.

Biopsy studies have demonstrated reductions in oxidative enzymic content of skeletal muscle and even in the structure and volume of mitochondria. There is even alteration in the fibre type distribution of muscle and a replacement of muscle fibres by fat, in addition to a marked loss of muscle bulk. Although chronically impaired blood flow may contribute to these muscle changes, some aspect of the neurohormonal imbalance of this syndrome seems more likely to lead to the catabolic state underlying the development of muscle wasting which, in severe cases, produces cardiac cachexia.

The only treatment which has been definitely shown to correct these metabolic abnormalities is physical exercise conditioning of the muscle[21], either localised or general, although some of the benefits of ACE inhibitors may be because of a chronic improvement in skeletal muscle blood flow.

Neuro-endocrine systems

Although initially supporting the failing heart, many of the body's compensatory mechanisms may prove harmful in the long-term[22]. This is particularly true for the neuro-endocrine systems and the autonomic nervous system. The initial response to a reduction in cardiac function is similar to that seen after blood loss: there is activation of the sympathetic nervous system, the renin-angiotensin-aldosterone system, and the vasopressin system, as well as reduction in vasodilator influences and in vagal tone.

All of these changes may be harmful if maintained chronically. Unopposed, angiotensin II, aldosterone and sympathetic activation cause intense vasoconstriction which further increases the after-load and work of the failing heart, as well as exacerbating vital organ hypoperfusion. Both may lead to direct myotoxic effects, worsen ventricular remodelling and predispose to ventricular arrhythmias.

The natriuretic peptide system

In historical terms, the natriuretic peptide system and its importance in cardiovascular biology have been recognised only relatively recently. However, the enormous amount of research conducted over the past 15 or so years has shown the central pathophysiological roles of this system in CHF. The widespread neurohormonal activation seen at the onset of heart failure is initially compensatory, e.g. the renin-angiotensin-aldosterone (RAS) system is activated in response to renal hypoperfusion and acts to retain salt and water.

As with the RAS system, activation of the natriuretic peptide system is initially compensatory, the natriuretic peptides being powerful vasodilators.

A number of closely related natriuretic peptides - atrial natriuretic peptide (ANP), B-type natriuretic peptide (BNP) and C-type natriuretic peptide (CNP) - have been described. Although natriuretic peptide synthesis may occur in a variety of tissues, ANP and BNP are mainly released from the cardiac atria and ventricles respectively. The main site of production of CNP may be the vasculature.

ANP and BNP appear to be synthesised in response to myocardial stretch. Increased plasma levels are seen in a variety of pathological conditions and are particularly elevated soon after AMI[23] and in CHF[24]. Plasma levels are closely related to the degree of left ventricular systolic dysfunction, and inversely related to prognosis. Indeed, plasma natriuretic peptide levels are among the most powerful indicators of prognosis in CHF[24] and are increasingly utilised as such.

A number of other related uses have been described and are likely to become more widespread over the next 20 years. As well as in CHF, the natriuretic peptides are powerful prognostic markers after AMI and can also help in the diagnosis of suspected left ventricular systolic dysfunction. In the latter situation, natriuretic peptide levels are much better at ruling out, rather than diagnosing, systolic dysfunction. A further possible use is in guiding pharmacological therapy in CHF; plasma natriuretic peptide levels fall with appropriate treatment and outcomes may be improved for patients by utilising plasma level of N-BNP to guide titration of pharmacological therapy[25].

Just as their role in clinical practice remains to be clarified, any causative role of the natriuretic peptides in the progression of CHF is not clear. They may be more than simply a marker of the extent of LV damage or dysfunction and may function to promote healing after acute myocardial injury. Studies have indicated that BNP facilitates infiltration of neutrophils into the infarct zone and may thus directly promote healing[26].

Potentially beneficial haemodynamic responses have recently been reported with nesiritide (recombinant human BNP) which has been used clinically to help manage decompensated heart failure[27]. However, doubts have been raised concerning the safety of this compound in clinical practice, and whether nestritide becomes a standard part of the management of such patients will have to await further reports.

The renin-angiotensin-aldosterone system

In untreated heart failure there is mild activation of the renin-angiotensin-aldosterone (RAS) system. This is dramatically augmented by the first therapeutic use of diuretics. The central importance of activation of the RAS to the pathophysiology of CHF is illustrated by the therapeutic benefit gained from the inhibitors of this system; angiotensin converting enzyme inhibitors, angiotensin receptor antagonists and most recently aldosterone receptor antagonists, can all improve prognosis in CHF.

All the components of the circulating RAS also exist in tissue sites. Activation of these local, tissue-based systems in the heart, kidney, brain and blood vessel walls is likely to be relevant in the pathophysiology of heart failure. The profound effects of ACE inhibition in delaying the progression of ventricular remodelling after a myocardial infarction (see Chapter Four) suggest that these systems are integral to the progression of heart failure.

The autonomic nervous system

An increase in sympathetic nervous tone and a concomitant reduction in resting vagal tone are seen early after a myocardial infarction, and are further increased in heart failure, especially after the addition of diuretics. The mechanism of persistent sympatho-excitation is not clear. The withdrawal of the chronic sympatho-inhibitory effects of the arterial baroreflexes is the common explanation, although this is a circular argument as sympathetic over-activity also directly leads to a reduction in baroreflex sensitivity.

Plasma noradrenaline, reduced baroreflex sensitivity and reduced heart rate variability all predict a poor prognosis in heart failure and all are markers of impaired sympatho-vagal balance.

Beta-receptor function

The chronic sympathetic over-activity described above has other adverse effects. Myocardial beta-1 receptor number and responsiveness is reduced in CHF, thought to be as a complication of persistent sympathetic stimulation. The importance of this may be in the resulting loss of myocardial responsiveness to sympathetic drive leading to an inadequate heart rate response to exercise (chronotropic incompetence) in addition to a loss of response to sympathomimetic stimulation.

Beta-receptor function may be directly relevant to the response to beta-blockade in heart failure. To date, only beta-blockers without intrinsic sympathomimetic activity have shown beneficial therapeutic effects in heart failure. Thus, the beneficial effect of these agents appears not to be a 'class effect'; one clinical outcome trial failed to show benefit from beta-blockade compared to placebo[28] and, indeed, one trial showed harm from the beta-blocker[29]. Thus the choice of beta-blocker for the management of CHF should be based upon demonstration of benefit from clinical trials.

The kidney

The kidney, central to salt and water homeostasis, is pivotal to the progression of heart failure. To a large extent, neuro-endocrine activation in heart failure is driven by relative hypoperfusion of the kidney. Reduction in renal perfusion pressure and increase in renal sympathetic nerve activity both reduce glomerular filtration and lead to clinically evident decline in renal function.

ACE inhibitors and angiotensin receptor blockers (ARB) have complex effects on the kidney, being protective in some patients but harmful in others. The presence of pre-existing renal disease, or the presence of renal artery stenosis are two factors which can predict an adverse response in renal function to the initiation of ACE inhibition or ARB. As any adverse effect of these agents on renal function is almost invariably reversible with reduction in dose or drug withdrawal, renal function should always be checked after commencing ACE inhibitor therapy. Moreover, where renal impairment is thought to be related to ACE inhibitors or ARB, lack of improvement in response to withdrawal of these treatments should lead to reconsideration of the diagnosis.

Fluid overload and hence oedema is common in heart failure, and electrolyte disturbances are both common and important. In mild heart failure fluid retention is due to the effects of aldosterone, vasopressin and catecholaminergic renal vasoconstriction. The kidney itself is also an active endocrine organ. In heart failure the juxta-glomerular apparatus, a specialised collection of neuro-endocrine tissue adjacent to the distal convoluted tubule, senses reduction in the rate of delivery of sodium to the distal tubule secondary to reduced renal blood flow.

In response the juxta-glomerular apparatus releases renin, thereby activating the circulating renin-angiotensin system. The resulting vasoconstriction further compromises cardiac output and renal perfusion leading to additional neuro-endocrine activation - this is the vicious cycle of heart failure.

All the components of the renin-angiotensin system also exist within the kidney and local autocrine activation of this system may have important effects on intra-renal haemodynamics. The vasoconstriction caused by the renin-angiotensin system is opposed by a second renal autocrine system, the kallikrein-kinin system. This system is also thought to be involved in the control of renal tubular function. Its precise role in heart failure and as part of the effects of angiotensin converting enzyme inhibitors (which also block the enzyme which breaks down bradykinin) is unknown.

In untreated heart failure there is initially retention of sodium and loss of potassium secondary to increased aldosterone levels. Later, particularly after loop diuretics have been given, there is further potassium loss. Eventually, hyponatraemia may occur, due to the unopposed effects of vasopressin and the use of high dose diuretics. Hyponatraemia is a very powerful adverse prognostic sign. Low magnesium levels can also occur in CHF and, together with hypokalaemia, may contribute to ventricular ectopy and more serious arrhythmias.

The Liver

In heart failure, the liver can be affected by elevated venous back-pressure and reduced nutritive blood flow. Increased venous pressure leads to hepatic congestion which may manifest clinically as abdominal discomfort, anorexia, nausea and vomiting. In severe cases ascites, intestinal malabsorption and malnutrition may occur together with impaired haemostatic function, hypo-albuminaemia and oedema.

Abnormal liver function tests are common in heart failure and are a marker of a poor prognosis. Pathologically, a centri-acinar pattern of fibrosis, often called cardiac cirrhosis, may be seen.

Table 2: **Complications of heart failure**

Arrhythmias	Atrial and ventricular brady- and tachyarrhythmias especially atrial fibrillation and ventricular tachycardia
Vascular	Peripheral emboli, postural hypotension
Renal	Renal impairment
Gastro-intestinal	Hepatic congestion and hepatic dysfunction, malabsorption
Musculoskeletal	Muscle wasting, abnormalities of histology, oxidative enzyme depletion, early fatigue
Respiratory	Pulmonary congestion, non-asthmatic bronchial constriction, respiratory muscle weakness, rarely pulmonary hypertension and right ventricular failure, sleep apnoea
Neurological	Increased incidence of stroke, fits and fainting

Summary

Although the reduction in cardiac function is the cause and central abnormality of heart failure, there is clearly a very wide range of abnormalities in other systems which contribute to both the symptoms and progression of the syndrome of CHF. Awareness of these changes aids the most appropriate use of the available therapeutic options to maximal effect. More effective novel treatment strategies await better understanding of the cause and effect of the non-cardiac abnormalities seen in the syndrome of CHF.

CHAPTER THREE

Treatment

Historical aspects

Historically, the treatment strategies used for heart failure have depended upon the prevailing knowledge of the pathophysiological basis of the disorder and how available pharmacological agents may modify it. As we have seen in Chapter Two, many disparate pathological processes occur in the syndrome of CHF.

Today we have a wide array of possible treatments, varying from inotropic agents to vasodilators, diuretics and agents which modify the neurohormonal response to heart failure. This was not always the case.

Early descriptions of heart failure can be found in the work of Hippocrates, including, it is interesting to note, a description of the non-cardiac pathology such as skeletal muscle wasting. At the time, the cause of the oedema and dyspnoea was not understood, but empirical therapies evolved probably by trial and error.

In the middle-ages most diseases were ascribed to alterations in the 'humours' of the body, and blood-letting or the use of herbal medicines was advised. The earliest description of the use of an agent we now know to be active was by William Withering over 200 years ago - the use of extract of foxglove containing digitalis alkaloids in the treatment of dropsy, a fair description of oedematous congestive heart failure. He described a 'cure' handed down by word of mouth by women versed in herbal medicines. This discovery was, of course, empirical, as was the use of quinine and later quinidine to suppress cardiac arrhythmias.

The first treatments chosen for their likely physiological effects were the mercurial diuretics, followed in the second half of the twentieth century by thiazide and loop diuretics, and then the modern treatment era. The evolution of these therapies was not entirely by chance. Major drug development now occurs almost entirely by screening new chemical entities for pharmaco-dynamic effects. By and large we can only find what we seek. Treatments for heart failure, therefore, will only be developed if they exert an effect thought to be of potential benefit in the treatment of heart failure.

Advances in understanding of the pathophysiology of the condition in the first half of the century focused on fluid accumulation, and hence diuretic agents were a logical first choice. Appreciation of weakening of cardiac contraction in heart failure led to screens for drugs with potentially useful positive inotropic actions. This helped to develop or discover the beta stimulants, other sympathomimetics and non-sympathomimetic inotropic agents including other cardiac glycosides, phosphodiesterase inhibitors and calcium sensitisers.

By and large these agents have failed to establish clear roles in the management of heart failure. Some have established roles in the support of the patient with cardiogenic shock but have proved very disappointing for longer-term management of CHF. This is partly due to the development of tolerance to their effects and partly due to increased mortality possibly related to pro-arrhythmic effects.

Agent after agent with the capacity to increase cardiac output and contractility has been shown to increase mortality, despite in some cases actually making the patient feel better and even improve exercise tolerance[30]. The only chronically administered positive inotropic agent safe to recommend in CHF is the original agent from 200 years ago, digoxin[31]. This is a sorry reflection of some of the non-success stories of modern pharmaceuticals.

The second major pathophysiological feature of heart failure to be addressed was the excessive vasoconstrictor drive, which impedes organ perfusion and adds to the loading conditions of the failing ventricle. Vasodilator medications are easily detected during drug development. Although controversial at first, there was soon a vogue for vasodilator therapy for heart failure. It improved symptoms and one regime, hydralazine with iso-sorbide dinitrate, was the first to suggest reduction in mortality in CHF patients[32]. No previous therapy had been shown in a controlled trial to have this effect. Other direct acting vasodilators followed, none of which have proved to be superior to this combination.

As will be discussed in Chapter Four, the ACE inhibitors proved to be a major advance in the use of vasodilator therapy in heart failure. First identified from the venom of a South American viper, ACE inhibitors were isolated and investigated because of a separate action; that of the inhibition of the kininase II enzyme leading to augmentation of bradykinin levels. This was the first discovered action of ACE inhibitors leading to their description as bradykinin potentiating factors (BPF). It was only realised much later that the same enzyme also converts angiotensin I to angiotensin II, and hence the major action of the ACE inhibitors was discovered only by chance.

There is still a school of thought that bradykinin accumulation may be as, or more, important than angiotensin conversion. ACE inhibitors were first used in the treatment of heart failure because of their vasodilator effects. There is now increasing evidence that vasodilatation per se may not be the most important effect of these agents. In inhibiting the production of angiotensin II and hence aldosterone, ACE inhibitors specifically block one aspect of the neurohormonal activation which is the hallmark of the body's response to heart failure. Additionally, ACE inhibitors partially block the sympathetic response as well.

This anti-neurohormonal action may be even more important than vasodilatation. This is supported by the findings of the second Veterans' Administration Heart Failure (V-HeFT II) study[33], which compared the ACE inhibitor enalapril to the hydralazine/isosorbide dinitrate regime which had been shown to be of value in the first V-HeFT study. The result was a greater reduction in mortality with enalapril despite a greater vasodilator effect with the other regime. These findings have led us to re-evaluate other strategies which inhibit the neurohormonal axis in heart failure; beta-blockers, more recently developed angiotensin II receptor blockers (ARBs), renin inhibitors, cardiac natriuretic peptides analogues, and endothelin antagonists.

More recently, selective blockers of angiotensin II on one of its receptors (the AT-1 receptor) have been developed. A number of these angiotensin II receptor blockers (ARBs) have been investigated for the treatment of heart failure. To date, these agents have been shown to be a suitable alternative in patients intolerant of ACE inhibitors[34] and to be equivalent to ACE inhibition in the context of post-MI LV dysfunction[35]. In select patients, largely those with advanced heart failure and limiting symptoms in spite of

ACE inhibitor and beta-blocker therapy, consideration may also be given to the addition of an ARB. Such an approach should be under specialist supervision and will be further discussed later.

As the ARBs, unlike the ACE inhibitors, do not block the enzyme kininase II they do not lead to a build up in bradykinin. Thus the ARBs are largely free of the major side-effect thought to be due to build-up of bradykinin, namely dry cough. As a result, some cardiologists use ARBs in patients intolerant of ACE inhibitors because of cough. There is no evidence that patients intolerant of ACE inhibitors for other reasons such as renal failure or severe hypotensive reactions are any more tolerant of the ARBs.

How many other potential treatments await discovery as we investigate more of the pathophysiology of this complex condition? The muscular, metabolic and endocrine abnormalities may also be valid targets for therapeutic intervention, as may reparative processes within the myocardium or more fundamental processes at the level of the myocyte.

We would need, however, to consider agents that do not have any acute cardiovascular effect at all, so we need to develop new screening procedures for potentially useful agents. An overview of the available treatment strategies for heart failure is presented in Table 3 (page 33).

Erythropoietin analogues

Anaemia is very common in heart failure. For example, in one small subset of the RENAISSANCE trial population, the prevalence of anaemia was around 12 per cent[36]. However, in studies of more typical heart failure populations, anaemia is more prevalent. In a recent study from our own institution, of patients hospitalised for the first time with heart failure, haemoglobin was below the World Health Organisation (WHO) parameters for anaemia (13.0 g/dl in men and < 12.0 g/dl in women) in 37 per cent of men and 43 per cent of women.

Anaemia is a strong prognostic indicator in heart failure[36]. Pilot studies regarding correction of anaemia in heart failure using erythropoietin have

Table 3: **Treatment options in the management of CHF**

General	• Salt restriction
	• Maintain optimal weight
	• Stop smoking
	• Encourage exercise
Specific	• Restrict excessive alcohol
	• Treat coronary risk factors
	• Control hypertension
Asymptomatic left ventricular dysfunction	• ACE inhibitor or ARB
Mild	• ACE inhibitor or ARB
	• Beta-blocker
	• Thiazide/loop diuretic +/-potassium supplements
	• Digoxin if in atrial fibrillation
Moderate	• ACE inhibitor or ARB
	• Beta-blocker
	• Loop diuretic +/- potassium sparing diuretics
	• Aldosterone antagonist
	• Consider combining ACE I and ARB
Severe	• ACE inhibitor or ARB
	• Beta-blocker
	• Loop diuretic
	• Aldosterone antagonist
	• Consider combining ACE I and ARB
	• Consider digoxin
	• Combine diuretics of different modes of action
	• Cardiac resynchronisation therapy
Intractable Heart Failure	• Transplantation
	• Cardiomyoplasty/Aortomyoplasty
	• Implantable Mechanical Assist Device
	• Haemofiltration

shown encouraging results regarding improved prognosis[37]. Randomised clinical trials are in progress using erythropoietin analogues to correct anaemia in heart failure.

Non-pharmacological treatment

Patients and their families are often confused and bewildered by the term 'heart failure' which has many negative and frightening connotations. Time spent explaining some simple aspects of the physiology of heart failure, the body's compensatory mechanisms and how these lead to symptoms, will often result in much better compliance with medication and avoidance of episodes of decompensation.

Many patients can be taught how to monitor their body weight at home on a daily basis and can often adjust the dose of diuretics within pre-set limits to achieve improved control of fluid balance. Detailed instructions from dieticians, physiotherapists and specialist heart failure nurses may be able to achieve maintenance of a reasonable quality of life while avoiding multiple admissions to hospital.

Rest and exercise

In acute heart failure bed-rest is a time-honoured way to control symptoms and help relieve oedema. A period of rest can improve both renal blood flow and the natriuretic response to diuretics. This is presumably via a reduction in the level of stimulation of the sympathetic and renin angiotensin systems, and it is still a therapeutic strategy in widespread use today.

Conversely, there is little evidence that bed-rest is of any benefit in the treatment of chronic non-oedematous heart failure. Ten to 20 years ago there was a vogue for prolonged bed-rest in the treatment of CHF or dilated cardiomyopathy, but this was never tested in a properly controlled trial. More recent evidence has been accumulated of the benefits of carefully tailored exercise training programmes for patients with stable CHF [38, 40].

After physical training, improvements have been seen in exercise tolerance, skeletal muscle and respiratory function and in autonomic and neurohormonal balance, correcting many of the pathophysiological changes of heart failure described in Chapter Two[41]. In a patient with stable CHF, with no evidence of exercise-induced ventricular arrhythmias, regular exercise should be encouraged rather than prohibited. Studies are underway to establish the best training programmes for these patients and whether training has any effect on prognosis.

Diuretics

Diuretics remain the mainstay of the management of oedema in heart failure. In acute heart failure intravenous loop diuretics lead to a dramatic and rapid improvement in condition, and in almost all patients with moderate or severe heart failure diuretics will be essential for adequate symptom control. Concern has been expressed about potential adverse effects of diuretic agents including activation of the sympathetic and renin-angiotensin systems, but until an alternative mechanism for the control of oedema fluid is achieved there remains no viable alternative to the use of these agents.

Initially, in mild heart failure, the thiazide diuretics may be sufficient but in more severe heart failure one of the loop agents - frusemide, bumetanide or torasemide - will be necessary. These are very familiar agents, particularly frusemide, but there remains some confusion about the best mode of treatment with these agents. Frusemide and bumetanide both give an acute and relatively short-acting diuresis which some patients find disabling. Others actually prefer this, as they can time their outings to avoid periods of diuresis. The newer torasemide has a much more prolonged action over 24 hours and the increase in urine flow is said to be much less obvious to the patient.

Initially, 40mg of frusemide or its equivalent (about 1mg of bumetanide) may be sufficient to control oedema, but some patients will need much higher doses of loop diuretics (frusemide 80 or 120mg bd.) for oedema control. A better alternative to increasing the dose of loop diuretic is to use combination diuretics by adding in agents of a different mode of action such as amiloride, thiazides or spironolactone, or all three together. This is often far more effective than even extremely high dose intravenous loop diuretics.

The potassium-sparing agents have the added advantage of ameliorating the loss of potassium produced by the other agents. As the majority of patients will be taking either ACE inhibitor or ARB, this is less of a problem than previously (for details of the use of ACE inhibitors, please see the next chapter). In an acute exacerbation, increase in oral dosing, switching to intravenous administration, or addition of a second (or third) class of diuretic can boost response.

Diuretic therapy should go hand in hand with sodium and fluid restriction. The 'Chinese take-away syndrome' is where an episode of acute pulmonary oedema occurs several hours after a high sodium meal in a previously stable CHF patient, due to the effects of acute sodium load and water retention. This should remind us of the effects of excessive sodium intake.

This can also be a problem with foreign travel where more restaurant meals are taken than usual, with a resultant and unpredictable increase in sodium intake. In severely affected patients fluid restriction may be necessary, but care should be taken not to produce dehydration and further deterioration in renal function. In the long-term, fluid restriction should not be to less than 1500ml per day.

A special note should also be made about metolazone, a thiazide-like diuretic with an especially profound diuretic action when given on the background of loop diuretic therapy. This combination can provide considerably more profound diuresis than intravenous administration of frusemide alone, even in high doses. As little as 2.5 or 5mg of metolazone given in this way can lead to several litres of extra urine output.

Profound electrolyte disturbance can accompany this diuresis. Metolazone should never be started for the first time in an outpatient, and should be reserved for specialist hospital use, except under special instruction. A small number of outpatients with severe oedematous heart failure require chronic administration of metolazone but often only 2.5mg on alternate days or once or twice a week may be needed. Care should be taken to monitor electrolytes, urea and creatinine very carefully in patients so treated.

Digoxin

Digoxin is the oldest drug therapy available for heart failure and it still retains a place as the only safe chronically administered positive inotropic agent.

Digitalis alkaloids have potentially serious side-effects, and also possess a narrow therapeutic window. In the presence of low potassium levels there is an increased possibility of serious ventricular arrhythmias. Its use in patients with rapid and poorly controlled atrial fibrillation is not controversial and this remains its main use in the UK. In patients with atrial fibrillation, 250 mg per day is a standard dose which should be reduced in the elderly, those with poor renal function or in patients with a low skeletal muscle mass, as it is heavily bound to muscle. Serum levels should be monitored regularly because of the narrow therapeutic window of digoxin and its potential for side-effects. It is the only available anti-arrhythmic agent which is not only free of negative inotropic effects but may actually possess chronic positive inotropic effects.

Its use in patients with sinus rhythm remains controversial, for although it is considered as first line standard therapy in the US and many European countries, cardiologists in the UK point to the lack of any prospective, placebo-controlled trial data demonstrating its long-term benefits in CHF with sinus rhythm. The 'DIG' trial compared digoxin and placebo on the background of standard heart failure treatment in 6800 patients and although there was no difference in mortality, the rate of hospitalisation appeared to be lower on digoxin[31]. Digoxin appears, therefore, to be safe in heart failure, although whether it is very effective remains controversial. Thus the indications for digoxin in CHF, in the absence of atrial fibrillation, are limited to the attempt to reduce re-hospitalisation in patients for whom such events are frequent.

Direct-acting vasodilators

As mentioned above, the major agents in this class in regular use for heart failure are the combination of hydralazine and isosorbide dinitrate.

Although an advance at the time, their use has been largely supplanted by the more effective ACE inhibitors.

Other agents such as prazosin have proved less effective, and the calcium antagonist vasodilators, particularly the short-acting dihydropyridine group, such as nifedipine, are significantly negatively inotropic and can worsen heart failure.

Some of the newer, longer acting agents, such as amlodipine or felodipine, may be safer and more effective. Amlodipine in particular has been shown to be safe and it may even reduce mortality in the subset of patients with heart failure without coronary disease. This comment is the result of a sub-set analysis and, as a result, is less reliable statistically. We cannot assume this effect of amlodipine has been proven.

Beta-receptor modifying agents

Manipulation of the cardiac sympathetic receptor system in CHF is an interesting therapeutic area; everything from pure beta-receptor antagonists e.g. metoprolol, through partial agonists (xamoterol) to pure beta-receptor agonists, has been tried or suggested for the treatment of heart failure. The present status is that beta-receptor agonists, although supporting the circulation acutely, have adverse chronic effects including loss of responsiveness, precipitation of ventricular arrhythmias and the worsening of beta-receptor down-regulation, which already occurs in CHF. The partial agonist xamoterol was bedevilled by similar draw backs, was associated with increased mortality in severe heart failure and, as a result, is no longer used in the management of CHF[29].

Beta-blockers

Despite the obvious problems of acute precipitation of heart failure in some patients, beta-blockers have received some support for use in carefully selected patients with heart failure for many years. For instance, an unexpected finding of the B-blocker Heart Attack Trial (BHAT) was that the major benefit of propranolol after acute MI was in patients with transient heart failure. In the last few years several large trials have shown benefits, in terms of both mortality and reduced hospital admissions, with a number of beta-blockers in CHF; carvedilol[42, 43], bisoprolol[44], metoprolol XL[45] and, most recently, nebivolol[46], have each shown useful therapeutic effects.

The use of beta-blockers in heart failure is complicated by intolerance and the precipitation of worsening of heart failure in a proportion of patients. However, as experience is gained, concerns are easing regarding the initiation and continuation of beta-blockers. It is important to remind ourselves that heart failure is characterised by a high frequency of repeated hospital admissions. The use of beta-blockers reduces the likelihood of hospital admission rather than making this more likely.

The initiation and titration of beta-blockers should take place under the supervision of professionals with experience of all aspects of the management of heart failure. The adage 'start low and go slow', suggesting initiation at low dose and slow, upwards dose titration, is the best approach to take. The patient should be counselled that they may experience some exacerbation of their symptoms (oedema, dyspnoea) soon after initiation or titration of beta-blocker.

Patients with heart failure are increasingly involved in the management of their own condition and can often be advised to manipulate their diuretic therapy, or to slow the rate of upwards titration of the beta-blocker. When carried out with care, a majority of patients with heart failure can be established and maintained on beta-blocker therapy.

There is no consensus on how to deal with an episode of worsening heart failure in a patient already on beta-blockade. Many cardiologists take the view that if, during acute exacerbation, the patient's heart rate is appropriate to the situation, i.e. the patient has a tachycardia, then the beta-blocker is unlikely to be responsible for the episode. The efficacy of these agents in the long-term management of heart failure is so well established that their continuation should be encouraged. My own practice is to try to continue the beta-blocker when at all possible.

Anti-arrhythmic therapy

Ventricular arrhythmias are extremely common in heart failure patients. It is important to remember that arrhythmias in heart failure are a manifestation of altered structure and disruption of normal electrical conduction in the myocardium. Those pharmacological agents that are associated with improved outcome in heart failure appear to achieve this at least partly through reducing the incidence of sudden death. This has been shown for ACE inhibitors and ARBs[34, 35], beta-blockers[44, 45] and aldosterone antagonists[47, 48].

As sudden death is common in heart failure, it is tempting to think that antiarrhythmic therapy, which can suppress the ventricular arrhythmias, may reduce the incidence of sudden death. Unfortunately, this approach has been ineffective; indeed, many anti-arrhythmic agents appear to increase the likelihood of sudden death.

Anti-arrhythmic agents should be selected with care where left ventricular function is known to be impaired. For atrial fibrillation, digoxin is safe and, as discussed above, may benefit some patients. Care should be exercised in paroxysmal atrial fibrillation.

A previous study suggested d-sotalol increased the likelihood of death in patients with AF and impaired LV function. Verapamil is negatively inotropic and is best avoided where LV function is impaired. Amiodarone is effective in suppressing both atrial and ventricular arrhythmias and has been studied in heart failure.

The GESICA trial, from South America, included a high proportion of patients with Chagas' cardiomyopathy and suggested amiodarone to reduce mortality in heart failure patients, regardless of the presence of ventricular arrhythmias. Subsequent trials in ischaemic left ventricular dysfunction failed to confirm this early promise[49, 50]. Indeed, a very recent trial showed amiodarone to have no effect on outcome in CHF, this being in distinction to the clear benefit afforded by the implantable cardioverter-defibrillator device[51]. Currently, these devices are indicated for patients with significantly impaired LV function who have survived documented ventricular arrhythmias.

Benefit has also been shown in the group of patients with significantly impaired function following acute MI, even without documented arrhythmias. In many health care systems, including the UK, the cost-effectiveness of this strategy is questionable and the main limitation to the use of these devices is their high initial and ongoing maintenance costs.

Any consideration to implantation of a cardioverter-defibrillator must be made under the care of a specialist. However, receipt of the device brings with it a number of issues for the patient; the knowledge that the device may deliver a shock can be difficult for the patient to deal with. Even more difficult for the patient can be the experience of actually receiving shocks from the defibrillator. These are usually appropriate and may be multiple. Patients should be counselled at length regarding the implications of implantation of such a device.

Oral positive inotropic agents

This group of drugs, including the phosphodiesterase inhibitors and calcium sensitisers, were supported as major advances when introduced into practice. However, trial after trial comparing them against placebo has shown not only loss of effect with time but has also suggested an increased mortality. Confusingly, one agent showed reduced mortality at one dose, and increased mortality at another[52].

Flosequinan, an agent initially thought to be primarily a vasodilator, was also associated with increased mortality, possibly due to pro-arrhythmic effects. With the exception of digoxin no safe chronically administered positively inotropic agent has been developed.

Anticoagulants and anti-platelet agents

There is clear evidence for the benefits of aspirin or other anti-platelet agents in patients recovering from a myocardial infarction. In the developed world, as the most common aetiology of heart failure is ischaemic heart disease, it is likely the majority will be treated with aspirin to reduce the chance of coronary arterial occlusion.

Some studies suggest that aspirin may attenuate the benefits of ACE inhibitors in heart failure[53]. However, a number of studies, including meta-analyses, failed to find evidence for this. Another possible indication for aspirin is in the prevention of cerebral embolism in chronic atrial fibrillation in patients with significantly impaired left ventricular function. Several studies have shown a positive effect of aspirin in this situation, although it's probably less profound than warfarin.

However, heart failure is associated with increased risk of cerebral thrombotic events even for those patients with sinus rhythm. But in clinical practice many patients are (very) elderly, and have one or more significant comorbidities which make the use of warfarin difficult. Full anticoagulation is usually reserved for those with heart failure who also have chronic or regularly recurrent atrial fibrillation, who have suffered a prior thrombotic or embolic stroke, or who suffer from transient ischaemic attacks.

CHAPTER FOUR

ACE inhibitors and angiotensin receptor antagonists

Introduction

The introduction of ACE inhibitors has had a profound effect on the treatment of cardiovascular disease. This is as true for heart failure as in any other area. ACE inhibitors, and more recently ARBs, have been studied rigorously in prospective placebo-controlled trials which have shown highly significant benefits with regard to symptoms, exercise tolerance and survival.

The benefits of ACE inhibitors are not restricted to patients with end-stage heart failure, but extend also to patients with mild to moderate heart failure, and even to modifying the progression of the disease in patients with asymptomatic left ventricular dysfunction.

This chapter will concentrate on the remarkable achievements made in documenting the role of ACE inhibition in the management of heart failure and its precedents. To this we will add the information from recent trials which indicate that the angiotensin receptor blockers (ARB) are an effective alternative to ACE inhibition in heart failure.

ACE inhibitors in severe heart failure

It is the unfortunate fate of many new pharmaceutical agents that they are tested first in the most hopeless situation. When the ACE inhibitor enalapril was trialled in this situation, in patients with severe CHF, a remarkable reduction in mortality was achieved.

In the CONSENSUS I study[54], 253 patients were randomly allocated to enalapril or placebo. Despite an overall six-month mortality in the placebo group of 44 per cent, there was a significant 40 per cent reduction in mortality in those randomised to enalapril. These patients were in end-stage heart failure, symptomatic at rest or on minimal effort. This treatment was a clear therapeutic breakthrough, so much so that almost immediately ACE inhibitors became standard therapy in this situation.

ACE inhibitors in mild to moderate heart failure

Within a few years of the CONSENSUS I study, similar evidence of benefit was shown for ACE inhibitors in the treatment of mild to moderate heart failure patients (New York Heart Association, NYHA class II and III) in whom moderate exertion lead to symptoms. The SOLVD treatment study[55] looked at 2569 patients with mild to moderate heart failure randomised to enalapril or control. One year mortality in these patients was 10-20 per cent rather than the 50 per cent or greater of the CONSENSUS I study patients.

Despite the lower overall mortality rate, enalapril again produced a significant 16 per cent reduction in mortality. Moreover, the ACE inhibitor was shown to be superior to the previous standard therapy. The V.HefT II study looked at 804 patients randomised between enalapril and the vasodilator combination, hydralazine/isosorbide dinitrate, and found a significantly lower mortality with enalapril (18 vs 25 per cent)[33].

ACE inhibitors in asymptomatic left ventricular dysfunction

It is known that there is poor correlation between objective measurements of left ventricular function and the degree of symptomatic impairment experienced by an individual patient. Moreover, patients with asymptomatic left ventricular dysfunction often develop symptomatic heart failure with time. Once the benefit of ACE inhibition had been proven in patients with advanced disease, attention turned to whether ACE inhibition could either delay the process by which asymptomatic disease progresses to clinical heart failure or indeed reduce mortality.

The prevention limb of the SOLVD trial[56], despite not showing any significant reduction in overall mortality, did show a reduction in the rate of progression of disease, with less new diagnoses of clinical heart failure. There was also a reduction in the rate of hospitalisation for heart failure suggesting that there may be both clinical and economic gains from the use of ACE inhibitors in this clinical situation.

The benefits are not as hard or clear-cut as the mortality reduction in symptomatic heart failure, and the patient group who may benefit are not as easily recognised because, by definition, they do not complain of symptoms. Thus the use of ACE inhibitors in these circumstances depends upon objective evidence of LV systolic dysfunction in the absence of symptoms. Most often this diagnosis occurs in the context of the patient having an echo for a reason other than symptoms suggestive of heart failure following MI, after the detection of LV hypertrophy on the ECG, or for the investigation of a cardiac murmur. As a result, ACE inhibitors have not become standard therapy in this situation but the use of these agents is increasing, i.e. very few patients are not prescribed ACE inhibition after MI. The use of ACE inhibitors in this situation is described below.

ACE inhibitors in patients recovering from a myocardial infarction

The area of infarcted myocardium does not form a stable scar immediately after the event, but rather undergoes a complex series of changes over weeks to months or even years. Some of these changes are beneficial and some are not. This process, known as ventricular remodelling, may hold some of the clues as to why patients can develop heart failure months or even years after a myocardial infarction without any evidence of further infarction.

In the first few days after the infarction, increased load on the residual myocardium leads to compensatory hypertrophy, partly stimulated by activation of some of the neurohormonal pathways described in Chapter

Two. The infarcted area is not protected from these influences. Over-stimulation of the adjacent myocardium by the sympathetic and renin-angiotensin-aldosterone systems can lead to even greater mechanical stress on the freshly infarcted region.

These processes can lead to the infarcted wall becoming stretched and thinned by the mechanical stress exerted upon it, and to an apparent increase in the extent of infarcted myocardium expressed in absolute size or as a percentage of the total left ventricular wall. This should be distinguished from infarct extension where previously living myocardium at the fringes of the infarcted area itself infarcts, leading to an increased size of wall motion abnormality.

Over time a second process may develop, where the wall of the whole myocardium becomes thinned and enlarged. This process affecting the residual myocardium involves re-alignment between myocytes, a process called cell slippage. This remodelling process leads to the ventricle enlarging and becoming progressively more globular in the absence of any further episodes of infarction.

Very good animal experimental data and observational data on patients have shown that this remodelling process precedes and predicts the development of heart failure months to years after an infarction.

Importantly, the remodelling process can be modified by interventions. The first large trial reported orally was the CONSENSUS II study[57]. Therapy was commenced with intravenous enalaprilat within 24 hours of the infarct and included subjects with quite low blood pressures at entry. The trial was terminated early with a non-significant trend towards an adverse effect on mortality when enalapril was given to relatively high-risk patients recovering from infarction.

This trial was rapidly followed by the SAVE trial which studied captopril in a target dose of 50mg tds in patients recovering from a myocardial infarction[58]. Unlike the CONSENSUS II study, the patients were recruited after the initial infarct healing phase had been completed, after most infarct expansion and scar formation had begun, but before the later remodelling process had become established. Investigations prior to trial entry included documentation of significantly impaired LV function by radionuclide ventriculogram ejection fraction of 40 per cent or less. In addition, all patients had undergone correction of clinically important residual myocardial ischaemia by either angioplasty or bypass surgery prior to entry to the trial.

Three to 16 days after infarction, 2231 patients were randomised to captopril or placebo and followed for 42 months. After the first six months of follow-up the survival curves for the two groups separated and, at the end of the trial, there was a significant 19 per cent reduction in total mortality. This mortality reduction was accompanied by a 22 per cent decrease in the rate of hospitalisation for heart failure.

Confirmation of the SAVE results followed rapidly. The AIRE study[59], co-ordinated from Leeds, recruited 2006 patients with clinical evidence of transient heart failure after acute myocardial infarction. This could include X-ray evidence of pulmonary oedema, or the presence of pulmonary rales, or a third heart sound on clinical auscultation. Patients were randomised to ramipril (5mg bd) or placebo between three and 10 days post-infarction. Ramipril treatment was associated with a significant 27 per cent reduction in mortality at 15 months of follow-up. The survival benefit appeared to commence in the first few weeks of follow-up. Similar beneficial effects in patients with large infarcts have also been shown for trandolapril.

Two further trials addressed the issue of whether ACE inhibitors could be beneficial in a wider cross-section of patients suffering myocardial infarction. These later trials recruited patients recovering from myocardial infarction irrespective of the presence or absence of clinical evidence of heart failure or objective evidence of LV dysfunction. The GISSI-3 trial of 18985 patients compared lisinopril versus control in an open label design, and found a small but significant 11 per cent reduction in mortality at six months of follow-up after as little as six weeks of therapy[60].

The ISIS-IV trial was by far the largest trial of ACE inhibitors in this setting with a total of 54824 patients randomised[61]. Exclusion criteria only included low initial blood pressure, a clear indication to captopril or known contra-indication to ACE inhibitors. ISIS-IV confirmed the findings of GISSI-3; there was a significant six per cent reduction in total mortality after as little as four weeks of treatment.

The overwhelming conclusion from these studies is that ACE inhibitors beneficially affect the recovery process after a myocardial infarction and, in the longer-term, reduce mortality by preventing the progression to heart failure. A reasonable clinical implication is that all patients with a documented myocardial infarction could benefit from four to six weeks of ACE inhibitor therapy where initially tolerated and any who manifest either clinical heart failure or significantly impaired left ventricular function (ejection fraction less than 40 per cent) thereafter, should remain on ACE inhibitors long-term.

These patients will form the majority of those who develop heart failure under the age of 65 in the UK. Based on available evidence the vast majority of patients either with heart failure, or at high risk of developing heart failure, should be on long-term ACE inhibitor therapy. These large trials have shown benefits in patients post-infarction and in those with established CHF, with a variety of ACE inhibitors, including enalapril, captopril, ramipril, lisinopril and trandolapril.

While it would seem a reasonable conclusion that the benefit of the ACE inhibitors is largely a class effect, we should take care regarding the dose of the individual agent chosen. Moreover, after MI, there is no good reason to choose to prescribe an individual ACE inhibitor which has no evidence of benefit in this situation.

Angiotensin receptor antagonists after myocardial infarction

As we have already mentioned, side-effects limit the use of ACE inhibitors in a significant proportion of patients. The most common events are renal impairment and cough, the latter most commonly leading to withdrawal of ACE inhibitor therapy. While the incidence of renal impairment is similar with ACE inhibitors and ARBs, the latter agents have an incidence of cough similar to that of placebo.

Moreover, long-term ACE inhibitor therapy is associated with a phenomenon called 'angiotensin escape', whereby plasma angiotensin II levels gradually increase to pre-treatment levels. This phenomenon may be associated with loss of benefit. Due to their mode of action at the angiotensin II (type I) receptor, this is not seen with ARBs. Freedom from cough led to studies of the potential use of ARBs as an alternative to ACE inhibitors after MI; freedom from angiotensin escape led to studies of the addition of an ARB to an ACE inhibitor.

The first study to compare these classes in the context of acute myocardial infarction was OPTIMAAL (Optimal Treatment In Myocardial infarction of the Angiotensin Antagonist Losartan)[62]. Comparing captopril 50mg tds to losartan 50mg od, this trial failed to demonstrate superiority of the ARB; indeed, it failed to show even non-inferiority compared to the ACE inhibitor.

A subsequent trial, VALIANT, had sufficient patients and end-points to compare three regimens: captopril 50mg tds, valsartan 160mg bd, or a combination of captopril 50mg tds plus valsartan 80mg bd[35]. There are two main results of VALIANT. Firstly, these three treatment regimens were associated with very similar outcomes - there was no additional benefit from combining ACE inhibitor and ARB. Secondly, the combination of ACE inhibitor and ARB was significantly less well tolerated than either agent alone.

To date valsartan is the only ARB with proven efficacy post-MI. Overall, we can say that this agent is an appropriate alternative to ACE inhibition in this setting, and that there is no gain from combining the drug classes. We can also say that the ARB losartan has been shown to be not as effective as ACE inhibition. Current practice is to use ACE inhibitors as the first-line choice after MI and, if not tolerated, to switch to an ARB. We should remember that for an individual patient, ACE intolerance due to renal impairment is likely to occur also with an ARB.

Angiotensin receptor antagonists in chronic heart failure

With regard to patients with established CHF, the effects of a number of ARB agents have been investigated. The largest such trial, the CHARM programme (Candesartan in Heart Failure Assessment of Reduction in Mortality and Morbidity) assessed the therapeutic effects of the ARB candesartan in three distinct groups of patients: (i) in patients intolerant of

ACE inhibition - the CHARM Alternative trial[34], (ii) as an add-on therapy in patients established on ACE inhibitor therapy - the CHARM Added trial[63], and (iii) in patients with heart failure in whom LV ejection fraction is preserved - the CHARM Preserved trial[64].

The CHARM Alternative trial randomised 2028 patients with heart failure and LV ejection fraction <40% to receive placebo or candesartan 32mg once daily. Mean LVEF was 30%, and 60% had a history of MI. Candesartan was associated with an approximately 23% reduction in the likelihood of death or hospitalisation for heart failure, a statistically highly significant result.

In the CHARM Added trial, 2548 patients with LVEF <40% and receiving ACE inhibitor were randomised to receive candesartan 32mg or placebo once daily. The patients in this arm of the CHARM programme were a population with quite advanced heart failure - mean LVEF was 28%, and over 70% had NYHA class III symptoms, i.e. dyspnoea on minimal exertion. In spite of this, the addition of candesartan was associated with a 15% reduction in the likelihood of cardiovascular death or heart failure hospitalisation. It is important to note that over 55% of patients in CHARM were being treated with a beta-blocker, reflecting contemporary practice.

Importantly, the tolerability of candesartan when given as an alternative to ACE inhibition is excellent. Thus, there is unequivocal evidence (from CHARM Alternative) that the ARB candesartan represents an excellent alternative to ACE inhibition in CHF. Moreover, we can say that in patients with marked symptoms in spite of current ACE inhibition and beta-blocker therapy, addition of candesartan may be appropriate.

At this point it is perhaps appropriate to consider the dilemma posed by the patient who, in spite of appropriate diuretic, ACE inhibitor and beta-blocker therapy, remains significantly symptomatic with restricted exercise capacity. In such a patient consideration should be given to additional pharmacological therapy. As noted above, we have evidence for some additional benefit from the addition of candesartan in this situation. Later we will see that addition of the aldosterone antagonist spironolactone in such patients is also associated with therapeutic benefit.

To date, no trial has compared the addition of candesartan (or any other ARB) with addition of spironolactone. Either agent may provide benefit but there is no direct evidence that either option is superior. It is appropriate to consider any patient who remains significantly symptomatic in spite of appropriate ACE inhibitor and beta-blocker, for expert review by a heart failure specialist - the combination of either ARB or spironolactone with ACE inhibitor therapy can be associated with a significant incidence of adverse effects.

CHAPTER FIVE

Initiating therapy for heart failure in a primary care setting

Introduction

The management of heart failure is increasingly becoming the joint responsibility of secondary and primary care. The diagnosis of heart failure often takes place at the first hospital presentation, whether this be with acute pulmonary oedema, dyspnoea, or in the context of acute myocardial infarction. Management strategies are increasingly aimed at reducing hospitalisation events; in many areas, heart failure nurse specialists are playing a pivotal role in achieving this goal. As such services become established, the aim will be to advance the detection and treatment of heart failure to an earlier stage of the disease.

The dramatic benefits shown for ACE inhibitors/ARB agents and for beta-blockers in all stages of left ventricular dysfunction make the early detection and treatment of this condition of utmost importance. Moreover, it is important to remember that all the major pharmacological classes that improve life expectancy in heart failure also reduce rehospitalisation. This is true for ACE inhibitors, ARBs, beta-blockers and aldosterone receptor antagonists. All clinicians involved in the management of CHF must be familiar with strategies for introducing and managing what have become standard pharmacological agents.

However, for many patients, the management of heart failure is becoming increasingly complex. The recent advent of aldosterone receptor antagonists and of cardiac resynchronisation therapy and implantable cardioverter defibrillator devices to the therapeutic regimen of many heart failure patients means that specialist knowledge and management is often required.

Detecting heart failure

On the one hand, detecting heart failure is one of the simplest and, on the other hand, one of the most complicated of clinical decisions. The patient with a massive myocardial infarction and acute pulmonary oedema holds little diagnostic difficulties to any practitioner; the elderly patient with insidious onset fatigue may not present or be recognised as having heart failure until the condition is advanced.

Moreover, an erroneous label of heart failure is often placed on a patient with idiopathic or venous peripheral oedema or breathlessness from non-cardiac disorders. Less usual symptoms for the presentation of heart failure include nocturia, urinary frequency, or chest discomfort. Cardiomegaly on a chest X-ray requested for another purpose may raise suspicion of heart failure.

The most important factor in detecting heart failure is a high index of suspicion. The doctor should seek evidence of left ventricular impairment and seek evidence of alternative diagnoses such as chronic lung disease, obesity, idiopathic or venous oedema, anaemia, muscular or neuromuscular disorders or psychogenic dyspnoea.

The signs detectable on clinical examination of acute and chronic heart failure are listed in Table 4, as well as the examination findings that may help in identifying the underlying cause. It must always be remembered that heart failure is not a diagnosis but a clinical syndrome. An underlying cause should always be sought, by clinical examination and further investigation including, where appropriate, referral to hospital.

Table 4: **Clinical examination findings in acute and chronic heart failure**

1. Acute heart failure	• Displaced and forceful apex beat • Third and/or fourth heart sound • Functional mitral or tricuspid regurgitation • Tachycardia • Low volume pulse • Right ventricular heave • Fluid retention: oedema, raised JVP, lung crepitations, liver congestion • Signs of impaired perfusion: cold, clammy skin, low blood pressure
2. Chronic heart failure	Can include all the signs of acute heart failure above, in addition to: • Skeletal muscle wasting • Cardiac cachexia • Cheyne-Stokes respiratory pattern
3. Signs of an underlying disorder	• Primary cardiac valvular disease, e.g. aortic stenosis • Atherosclerotic vascular disease • Severe hypertension • Signs of severe anaemia or volume overload, e.g. A-V shunt • Significant arrhythmia • Evidence of generalised myopathy or poisoning

Investigating heart failure

A detailed history, physical examination and interpreted ECG will identify the underlying disease process causing heart failure in the majority of cases. There remains a significant proportion in whom an initial cause cannot be found. Heart failure should not be accepted as a diagnosis without identification of its aetiology; neither should a diagnosis of idiopathic cardiomyopathy be accepted until reasonable lengths have been pursued to exclude alternative diagnoses, as some underlying causes are treatable in their own right. In particular, previously undetected ischaemic heart disease should be considered.

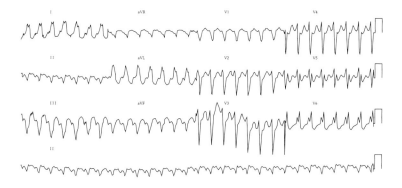

*Figure 5.1 – **The ECG at presentation to hospital of a 60-year old male complaining of shortness of breath. Cardiovascular risk factors included hypertension and a positive history of coronary artery disease. The ECG shows atrial flutter with 2:1 atrioventricular conduction, and a left bundle branch block QRS morphology. He failed to cardiovert with pharmacological intervention but did so on insertion of a urinary catheter. Echocardiography at this stage showed global impairment of LV function. The working diagnosis was idiopathic dilated cardiomyopathy.***

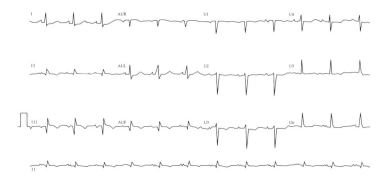

Figure 5.2: **The ECG after cardioversion. This shows Q-waves in the inferior leads, 1st degree heart block and atrial hypertrophy. In spite of there being no history of MI, or indeed of chest pain, coronary arteriography showed totally occluded right coronary artery (in keeping with the inferior Q-waves), significant left coronary artery and circumflex artery stenoses. The inferior wall of the myocardium was akinetic, and the anterior wall very hypokinetic, with overall LV ejection fraction around 25%.**

This was in fact a case of ischaemic cardiomyopathy, and illustrates the importance of appropriate investigations in the diagnosis of the aetiology of heart failure.

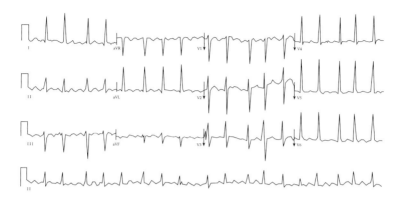

Figure 5.3: **Idiopathic dilated cardiomyopathy - the ECG of a 29 year old male presenting to hospital with four weeks of progressive dyspnoea. Examination revealed cardiomegaly and resting tachycardia. There was no evidence of pulmonary or peripheral oedema. The ECG shows atrial flutter and suggests left ventricular hypertrophy (tall R-waves in I. aVL, V4-V6; deep S-waves in III, V1-V2). Echocardiography showed biventricular dilatation and globally impaired function. The coronary arteries were normal.**

Essential investigations in all cases should include ECG, chest X-ray, biochemistry, thyroid function tests and full blood count. It is now accepted that all cases should have echocardiography to both confirm heart failure and to help identify the cause. Where no cause is immediately apparent, iron studies and calcium estimation may reveal a potentially treatable cause. Where the cause of the heart failure is not apparent, specialist referral should be the rule rather than the exception.

Referral may be necessary to obtain exercise electrocardiography or echocardiography, although in some cases these tests may be available to general practitioners or specialist nurses via an open access service. Exercise testing gives an objective measure of limitation and can detect significant ischaemic heart disease. Echocardiography will confirm the presence and severity of left ventricular dysfunction and often give good evidence for the cause. It will also detect and quantify the severity of suspected or unsuspected valvular diseases that may be the cause of the disorder. Other conditions such as pericardial effusion can also be detected.

Other, more specialised, investigations in cases still remaining undiagnosed include:

- cardiopulmonary exercise testing with analysis of respiratory gas exchange
- other imaging techniques such as radionuclide ventriculography
- cardiac magnetic resonance imaging
- echocardiographic or isotope imaging with pharmacological stress agents
- Holter monitoring
- cardiac catheterisation
- ventricular biopsy
- investigation for heavy metal poisoning and for endocrinopathies.

The circumstances of each case will dictate which of these investigations are ultimately required. A list of useful investigations is given in Table 5.

Assessing treatment for new cases of heart failure

New cases presenting with dyspnoea or fatigue with fluid retention should be prescribed a diuretic (thiazide or low dose loop diuretic, e.g. frusemide or bumetanide) and investigated initially with chest X-ray, ECG, biochemistry and blood count. Echocardiographic examination should be requested. The response to initiation of diuretic therapy should be checked within a few days and the diagnosis reconsidered. If the response to therapy has been as expected, further investigations to confirm the degree of LV dysfunction and its cause, should be initiated. If the response to therapy has not been as expected, the diagnosis should be reconsidered.

Table 5: **Useful investigations for the patient with chronic heart failure**

1. To detect heart failure	Echocardiogram: impaired left ventricular contraction
	Chest X-ray: increased cardiothoracic ratio, congestion
	Cardiopulmonary exercise testing: objective exercise tolerance, maximal oxygen uptake, ability to check limitation is cardiac (respiratory exchange ratio exceeds 1.0, no arterial oxygen desaturation or CO_2 retention) rather than respiratory (arterial oxygen desaturation or CO_2 retention) or non-cardiopulmonary (peak respiratory exchange ratio less than 1.0)
2. To look for underlying causes	ECG: ischaemia/infarction, LVH, arrhythmia
	Echocardiogram: valvular disease, systolic versus diastolic impairment
	Rare causes: hypocalcaemia, thyroid heart disease, iron storage diseases, anaemia, heavy metal poisons, amyloid (serum electrophoresis, rectal biopsy), sarcoid (serum ACE, Kveim test)
	Cardiac catheter and, rarely, ventricular biopsy
3. To assess severity	Radionuclide or angiographic ventriculography or echocardiography for ejection fraction
	ECG, QRS duration and morphology
	Cardiopulmonary exercise testing
4. For prognosis	Plasma natriuretic peptide levels
	24-hour Holter ECG monitoring for ventricular arrhythmias
	Blood tests useful for prognosis: haemoglobin, renal function, electrolyte and liver disturbances

Early hospital referral should be considered for:

- younger patients
- all cases with concomitant angina
- those with significant valvular heart disease
- those with severe heart failure
- those not responding to diuretic therapy appropriately.

At the follow-up visit the dose of diuretic should be reviewed after assessing the response and the patient's present fluid status.

Once the diagnosis of heart failure due to systolic left ventricular dysfunction has been made, the introduction of an ACE inhibitor should be considered. The cause of heart failure will usually be evident from the clinical history (previous myocardial infarction, hypertension, valvular heart disease), ECG (old myocardial infarction, left ventricular hypertrophy, arrhythmia), and basic laboratory investigations (anaemia, thyroid disease). In many cases echocardiography will provide additional information regarding aetiology.

Assessing treatment for pre-existing cases of heart failure

The evidence for the benefits of ACE inhibition (and for certain ARBs as an alternative) is so strong that we should seek out existing patients on diuretic therapy for heart failure and assess them for the introduction of ACE inhibitor therapy, even if they are well controlled and symptomatically stable.

Many practices now have computerised prescriptions records that will allow diuretic users to be identified and a review of the notes will determine whether these were prescribed for heart failure. We should go even further and reassess patients with known coronary artery disease especially those who have had a myocardial infarct in the past. This group may include many patients with significant left ventricular dysfunction and even unrecognised heart failure, a number of whom will have experienced their infarct prior to the advent of ACE inhibitor, and particularly beta-blockade, in heart failure.

Once identified, these patients should be re-evaluated in a similar way to new presentations. Evidence should be obtained about their symptoms, clinical signs and left ventricular function. If significantly impaired ventricular function is suspected, e.g. from cardiac enlargement, increased filling pressures on the jugular venous pulse, peripheral oedema, pulmonary oedema or an added heart sound, then they should have their diuretic dose reviewed, their biochemistry and blood count reassessed and ACE inhibitors commenced.

Open access echocardiography

General practitioners quite rightly desire access to the best diagnostic facilities to enable them to care for their patients, and feel they do not always need to involve the hospital specialist. The UK cardiologist feels that the provision of echocardiography is too limited to offer a free-for-all, and that the hospital echo service could not cope with the extra demand.

However, the vast majority of practitioners involved in the management of patients with heart failure agree that echocardiography is vital. Given the high cost of heart failure, the proven advantages of pharmacological therapy and the finding that lack of confirmation of heart failure by echocardiography is one of the reasons for physicians not commencing ACE inhibitor and other therapy, there is a strong argument that adequate echo facilities must be provided.

As suggested in the NICE guidelines document[65], echocardiography should be available for patients with suspected heart failure following consideration of the likelihood of the condition. This is assessed from the medical history, clinical examination, and consideration of the ECG. Probably the ideal service is a rapid access echo service with specialist input into the report and management recommendations that go with the report.

Initiating ACE inhibitor therapy

The concerns of all practitioners regarding initiation of ACE inhibitor therapy, particularly for primary care physicians and heart failure nurse specialists, are symptomatic hypotension and renal dysfunction. So-called 'first-dose hypotension' is a misnomer. In heart failure, the blood pressure response to a given dose of ACE inhibitor is very similar after chronic therapy and after the first dose.

What is important clinically is whether the blood pressure response is accompanied by symptoms; dizziness, pre-syncope, visual disturbance and excessive tiredness may be the manifestations of hypotension. The incidence of symptomatic hypotension requiring cessation of therapy is very low if simple precautions are taken and guidelines followed.

The patient at highest risk of symptomatic hypotension is the elderly patient already on high dose diuretics, who is dehydrated, has poor autonomic cardiovascular control and renal function and who is given a large initial dose of ACE inhibitor. Avoiding these circumstances makes ACE inhibitor initiation safe in general practice. Contrary to popular belief, patients with the highest pre-treatment blood pressure are likely to show the greatest fall. However, the extent of the blood pressure response bears little relationship to the likelihood of symptoms.

Fluid balance should be assessed and commencement of treatment avoided when the patient is dehydrated. While it is common practice to consider reduction in the dose of diuretics for 24 to 48 hours prior to initiation, there is very little evidence that this reduces the likelihood of symptomatic hypotension.

If the patient is moderately high-risk as defined by the factors listed above, it is advisable to commence dosing in the surgery or clinic with a low dose of a short-acting ACE inhibitor, such as 6.25mg captopril so that any hypotension will be limited and short-lived. The average blood pressure response to 2mg of perindopril is less than with some other agents in the class[66]. However, the range of blood pressure responses seen is very similar among ACE inhibitors[67], and the risk of symptomatic hypotension is always present.

If the patient does not fit into the high-risk group then a low initial dose of a longer-acting ACE inhibitor, such as 2.5 or 5mg lisinopril, can be given at bed-time so that the patient is supine without recent diuretic administration when the first dose is taken. Care should be exercised in this regard; many patients are elderly men troubled by nocturia in whom a pharmacologically induced nocturnal fall in blood pressure may present its own problems.

Figure 5.4: **Demonstrating a simple strategy for initiating the ACE inhibitor or angiotensin receptor blocker**

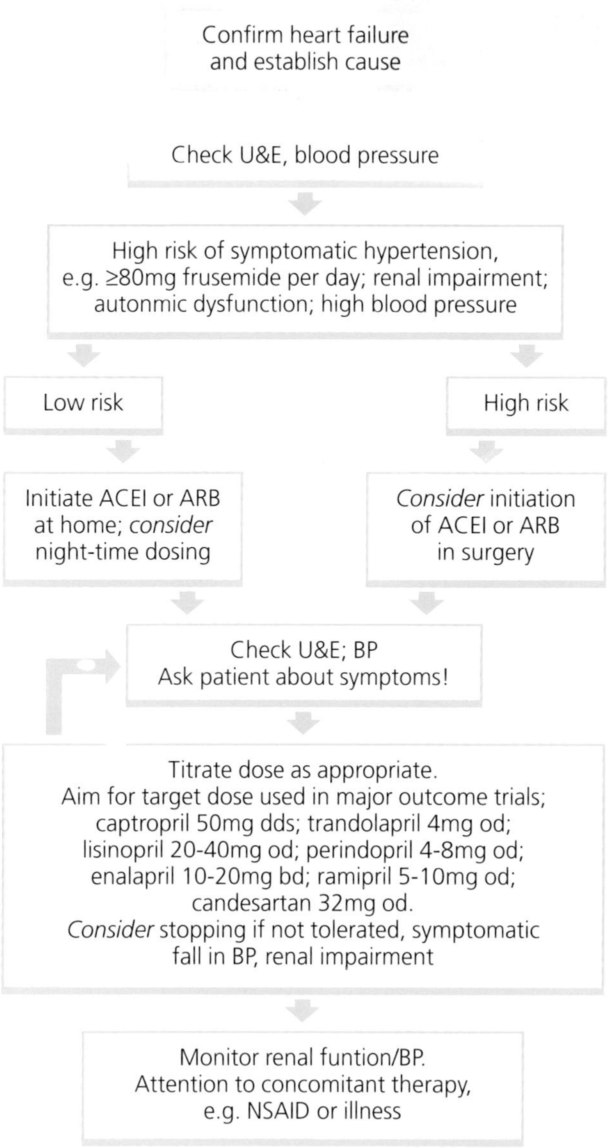

Confirm heart failure
and establish cause

Check U&E, blood pressure

High risk of symptomatic hypertension,
e.g. ≥80mg frusemide per day; renal impairment;
autonmic dysfunction; high blood pressure

Low risk

High risk

Initiate ACEI or ARB
at home; *consider*
night-time dosing

Consider initiation
of ACEI or ARB
in surgery

Check U&E; BP
Ask patient about symptoms!

Titrate dose as appropriate.
Aim for target dose used in major outcome trials;
captropril 50mg dds; trandolapril 4mg od;
lisinopril 20-40mg od; perindopril 4-8mg od;
enalapril 10-20mg bd; ramipril 5-10mg od;
candesartan 32mg od.
Consider stopping if not tolerated, symptomatic
fall in BP, renal impairment

Monitor renal funtion/BP.
Attention to concomitant therapy,
e.g. NSAID or illness

Choosing the correct dose

The doses of ACE inhibitors and ARBs given in practice for patients with heart failure are commonly far less than those shown in the major trials as having a beneficial effect on disease progression and life expectancy. Doctors are inherently cautious and would like to opt for a lower dose especially when some of the side-effects, such as hypotension, renal impairment and possibly cough, may be dose related.

For hypertension at least we have an intermediate therapeutic goal, that of blood pressure reduction, to assess the correct dose. In contrast, for heart failure, there is little we can measure to estimate whether our treatment is having an effect on outcome. As a result, we are uncertain whether to push up the dose and many practitioners settle for a lower dose. Trials comparing low-dose with high-dose ACE inhibition have suggested that higher doses are associated with relatively greater impact on outcome. The correct strategy is to increase the doses towards those used in the major trials and accept a lower dose only if a dose-related problem has occurred.

Currently, ACE inhibitors are the first choice for patients with heart failure, ARBs being reserved for those patients intolerant thereof. The side-effect profile of ARBs is better than for ACE inhibitors, largely due to the relative absence of the side-effect of cough. It is likely that, with time, we will see increasing use of ARB agents.

All of the above points regarding initiation of ACE inhibitor therapy in heart failure are equally applicable to initiation of ARB therapy. Other than for cough, the incidence of renal impairment, symptomatic hypotension, and hyperkalaemia are very similar with the two drug classes. If consideration is to be given to switching a patient from ACE inhibitor to ARB, there is little to support the strategy of stopping the ACE inhibitor and then slowly titrating the ARB from a low to high dose. It is reasonable to move directly from ACE inhibitor to ARB.

Initiating beta-blocker therapy

The current situation regarding initiation of beta-blockers is comparable to that which existed with ACE inhibitors a few years ago. For many years after their introduction, initiation of ACE inhibitor therapy was viewed with trepidation by many physicians in both primary and secondary care. Time, experience and the growing acceptance of the benefits of this therapy have largely dissipated these concerns. However, the concept of beta-blockade for heart failure is contrary to what most practising physicians were taught. Indeed, many physicians have first-hand experience of inducing acute pulmonary oedema as a result of their initiating beta-blockade. In addition, concerns are often raised regarding beta-blockers in patients with 'asthma' or peripheral vascular disease.

However, it must be emphasised that beta-blockade in heart failure is safe. Regarding 'asthma', reversible airways obstruction is a relative, rather than an absolute, contraindication to beta-blockade. It is, in reality, very rare to induce broncospasm with these agents. Moreover, many patients with a label of 'asthma' have irreversible airways obstruction or indeed dyspnoea which is not related to airways disease.

With regard to causing decompensation of heart failure, at its most florid presenting as acute pulmonary oedema, this can be avoided with the application of appropriate care. Beta-blockers should be initiated at a low dose and titrated upwards at intervals of a few weeks. Currently, two beta-blockers are licensed in the UK for the management of heart failure. Bisoprolol should be initiated at a dose of 1.25-2.5mg and titrated to a target dose of 10mg od. Carvedilol should be started at 3.125mg bd and titrated to a target of 25mg bd.

The use of carvedilol[42, 43] and bisoprolol[44] is based upon evidence from large-scale clinical trials. Recently, a third beta-blocker, nebivolol, has been shown to be associated with favourable effects on outcome in heart failure[46]. To date this agent is not licensed for the management of heart failure. As noted earlier, it cannot be assumed that the effect of beta-blockers in heart failure is a class effect; some beta-blockers have been associated with adverse effects in this condition.

As with ACE inhibitors or ARBs, initiation of beta-blockade may be associated with symptomatic fall in blood pressure. The question is often asked as to whether, in a newly diagnosed patient, the ACE inhibitor or the beta-blocker should be initiated first. Many cardiologists take the view that in the patient with concomitant angina or soon after MI, the beta-blocker is a logical first choice. This is very reasonable. We must also remember that beta-blockade should not be regarded as an alternative to ACE inhibition in heart failure. Other than for the patient intolerant of ACE inhibition and ARB therapy, beta-blockade should be an addition to one or other agent.

Initiation of aldosterone antagonist therapy

The pharmacological management of heart failure becomes ever more complex. In patients with advanced heart failure (NYHA functional class III or IV in spite of appropriate diuretic and ACE inhibitor therapy) the aldosterone receptor antagonist spironolactone is associated with improved outcome[47].

Similarly, in patients with LV dysfunction after MI, the aldosterone antagonist eplerenone has beneficial effects on mortality and hospitalisation[48]. This is on top of standard background therapy, including diuretic, ACE inhibitor / ARB and beta-blocker.

The use of these agents in heart failure should be under the care of a practitioner with experience in the management of heart failure and of these agents in particular. The evidence for these agents at the moment pertains to specific patient groups only. Both are associated with a significant incidence of hyperkalaemia and renal dysfunction.

CHAPTER SIX

Maintenance therapy, follow-up and referral needs, and new developments

Introduction

Chronic heart failure is a permanent disorder. The patient may be stable for many months or years, and be free of symptoms, but this does not represent a cure. The possibility of relapse and deterioration is always present and therapy should always be monitored to minimise the chances of such deterioration. Time should be spent with the patient and family to explain the nature of the condition, the action of the prescribed medicines and common reasons for episodes of decompensation, for this explanation may help to prevent some relapses into acute heart failure. The recognition of heart failure as a chronic disease elicits consideration of management strategies used in other chronic conditions.

Creating a care plan

For each patient after diagnosis and hospital assessment where appropriate, a care plan should be produced. This should be based on rational assessment of the needs for regular review, based on the likelihood of maintaining stable control of the patient's heart failure. The patient and family should be advised on the need for regular review rather than just the collection of repeat prescriptions, and the reasons for this should be explained.

Ideally, a heart failure nurse specialist should be intimately involved in formulating and implementing the management plan. Attempts should be made to target interventions to those at highest risk of hospitalisation; these patients are, by definition, those who have previously, indeed recently, been hospitalised with heart failure. Shared-care with a hospital specialist unit may be necessary and this should always be considered in the care plan.

The care plan should assess the frequency of review, measurement of urea and electrolytes and haemoglobin, the need for hospital assessment and the need for special monitoring, e.g. daily weighing at home, regular exercise, drug level for digoxin or other blood tests. If the patient knows these requirements then loss to proper follow-up will be less frequent.

The patient and family should be instructed in dealing with episodes of deterioration such as fluid retention, palpitation, episodes of chest pain, side-effects of drugs and when to call for assistance. Addressing these fears will pay off in the longer term with more stable patients and less calls of an emergency nature.

Where available, access to heart failure nurse specialists should be provided. Initially, for example after hospital discharge, this may entail home visits for monitoring of the patient's condition and serology. The frequency of such direct contact will in all likelihood reduce with time. Direct contact may eventually become unnecessary with time but the nurse service should always be available to the patient.

Primary care or shared care

For each patient, the nature of follow-up should be determined. In the younger patient, those with concomitant angina or severe failure, or those being considered for surgical therapies, regular hospital review will be necessary. In addition, some patients suffer episodes of deterioration necessitating hospital admission. It is better for these patients to see the hospital physician regularly, rather than just as crisis management when conflicting treatment strategies may lead to confusion and poorer long-term control.

The frequency of hospital follow-up and the distribution of care between the hospital and general practice should be discussed with the hospital consultant. Again, the heart failure nurse specialist can provide liaison and communication between all parties involved in patient management. For many, routine hospital outpatient visits are not necessary, but in others a properly designed shared care arrangement has considerable advantages.

Monitoring therapy

Every patient on diuretic and ACE inhibitor/ARB therapy should have regular urea and electrolyte monitoring at least once a year - often more frequently - and have their condition assessed at least every three months. Specialist investigations such as echocardiography may be necessary in selected patients on a regular basis in cases where significant silent deterioration may be occurring such as valvular heart disease, idiopathic dilated cardiomyopathy or in critical ischaemic heart disease.

Other tests such as exercise tests and advanced imaging tests may be needed, and these may justify regular hospital review. There is no point in a patient attending hospital outpatients every few months if nothing is done which cannot be done in general practice. This underlines the need for an agreed care plan among the hospital consultant, GP and heart failure nurse specialist to define the need for, and purpose of, regular specialist investigation.

Reasons for referral

It is not practical to refer all patients with heart failure to hospital, but as a life-long condition it would be appropriate to refer all patients who did not achieve control of symptoms after initial therapy. This may be only for initial diagnosis and for the preparation of a care plan. The indications for referral of CHF patients are listed in Table 6.

Table 6: **Reasons for referral to hospital**

1. Uncertain aetiology of heart failure

2. Young age
- Limiting symptoms in a young patient (<65 years) where specialist investigations and intervention may be indicated

3. Unexpectedly poor response to therapy

4. Potential for therapeutic intervention
- Co-existing angina indicating consideration of coronary revascularisation
- Valvular dysfunction indicating possible valve surgery
- Arrhythmias for drug therapy, pacemaker or implantable defibrillator
- Left bundle branch block and significant limitation of exercise capacity
- Potential transplant or myoplasty candidate

5. New or difficult therapies
- To commence ACE inhibition, beta-blockade in high risk patients
- To commence aldosterone antagonist therapy

6. Unstable or complicated patients
- Those with multiple admissions or episodes of decompensation
- Those requiring specialist paramedical help, dietician, physiotherapy, occupational therapy, palliative care and social work advice specific to the problems of end-stage heart disease

One of the major reasons for referral is to offer patients the most modern treatments for heart failure. The management of heart failure has progressed impressively over the last decade and even over the last few years. Busy general practitioners cannot expect to keep abreast of all new developments unless they have regular contact with a specialist heart failure unit.

New treatments are being developed for the management of heart failure patients and some of these are described briefly below. It should be remembered that today's advances were yesterday's novel treatments. A severely limited patient may gain considerable benefit from taking part in an early trial of a new therapy. There is considerable evidence that even taking part in a clinical trial leads to more careful management and better outcome regardless of the treatment given. The patient and family may need advice on the purposes, uses and advantages of taking part in clinical trials for heart failure.

Prognosis

Severe heart failure has a very poor prognosis with a one-year survival rate of 50 per cent or less. In mild to moderate heart failure it is approximately 20-30 per cent per year. Many separate parameters have been described as having prognostic value in patients with heart failure. It is important to differentiate between factors which have a direct functional link to increased mortality (and which might be amended to improve prognosis), and prognostic markers which merely reflect a worse prognosis.

Low ejection fraction, the degree of functional limitation, electrolyte disturbance, anaemia, renal dysfunction, the degree of neurohormonal or autonomic dysfunction and, to a lesser extent, the presence of ventricular arrhythmias, are all markers of an adverse prognosis. There are also general factors such as age or the presence of comorbid conditions which affect outcome.

Newer developments in the management of heart failure

Cardiac resynchronisation therapy (CRT)

Chronic heart failure is often associated with aberrant electrical conduction within the myocardium. This manifests itself as prolongation of the QRS complex on the ECG, often as a bundle branch block pattern. The prolongation of the ECG indicates slow, protracted electrical depolarisation of the myocardium. This results in slow, protracted and dys-synchronous myocardial contraction; there is dys-synchrony between atrial and ventricular contraction, and importantly between right and left ventricular contraction. In addition to mechanically inefficient myocardial work, this dys-synchrony often results in mitral regurgitation, compounding the patient's symptoms and cardiovascular status. Cardiac sys-synchrony impacts on functional status and on prognosis; indeed prognosis is inversely related to the QRS duration. A number of trials have investigated the effect of resynchronisation therapy; the right and left ventricles are simultaneously paced, as is the right atrium, to maximise ventricular filling.

A landmark trial, CARE-HF (Cardiac Resynchronisation in Heart Failure), reported recently and for the first time showed that CRT can impact favourably on life expectancy in patients with CHF. Patients were NYHA class III (75%) or IV (25%), mean LVEF was 25%, and QRS duration 160msec. Compared to best medical therapy, CRT was associated with an approximately 35% reduction in the combined end-point of all-cause mortality or unplanned cardiovascular hospitalisation. Indeed, the effect on all-cause mortality alone was similar.

CRT represents a major advance in the treatment options for advanced heart failure. However, the procedure is technically challenging, selection of patients can be difficult, and the cost is high. As with all management considerations in advanced, i.e. NYHA III or IV, heart failure, specialist opinion is required.

Rehabilitation

Heart failure is a life-long condition and the patient and family should be advised that a complete 'cure' is unlikely. Care should be taken, however, to demonstrate that the condition can be improved dramatically, and that it is not a sentence of either death or permanent disability. The use of exercise training has increased exercise capacity considerably in some patients (see Chapter 3) and it may be possible for patients with optimum therapy and a period of comprehensive rehabilitation to go back to meaningful employment.

Many rehabilitation schemes initially designed to deal only with post-MI or post-surgical patients are extending their services to patients with heart failure. Indeed, the nature of the symptoms in CHF lend themselves to exercise programmes akin to those used in pulmonary rehabilitation.

Coronary bypass graft surgery

Coronary bypass surgical techniques and myocardial preservation have improved significantly over the last few years. As a result, surgeons are operating on patients with more marked left ventricular impairment. The presence of heart failure need not preclude consideration of this procedure in patients with co-existing angina, as major symptomatic benefit could be obtained by relief of angina.

Hibernating myocardium and revascularisation

It has been recognised that in some cases of heart failure secondary to ischaemic heart disease, left ventricular function can be improved by procedures which increase the blood supply to the myocardium even in the absence of angina. Although there is uncertainty about the precise pathophysiological mechanisms which underlie this, there appears to be a phenomenon of so-called 'hibernation' where an area of left ventricular myocardium can be poorly or non-contracting, but which is still alive, and which can improve its contractile performance after revascularisation.

The evaluation of these patients involves identifying possible candidates: those with ischaemic heart disease and heart failure in excess of that suggested by the number or size of episodes of infarction. These patients need specialist investigation, including cardiac catheterisation and evaluation for hibernation of myocardium. This can be done by stress echocardiography, late uptake of thallium on radionuclide scans (indicating viable myocardium in a non-functioning region) or by PET scanning, indicating metabolic activity in an apparently infarcted area.

The choice of the revascularisation procedure between graft surgery or angioplasty will depend on the nature and extent of the coronary arterial disease.

Cardiac transplantation

This is an effective therapy for severe heart failure untreatable by other surgery or still limiting despite maximal medical therapy. The demand far outstrips the supply of organs so, unfortunately for many patients, there is a long wait for an operation. Consideration should be given to more severely afflicted patients, younger patients with more years to gain, and those in whom all other possibilities have been tried.

Cardiomyoplasty and aortomyoplasty

These are still experimental procedures. Skeletal muscle from the back, usually Latissimus Dorsi, is converted by appropriate electrical stimulation to a non-fatiguing muscle type and then wrapped around either the heart or the descending aorta to act as an assist pump stimulated at appropriate points in the cardiac cycle to augment myocardial contraction. It shows some promise and is being tested in major heart failure surgical units.

Stem-cell therapy

The theory of this approach, currently experimental, is that stem cells from a given patient may potentially differentiate into functional myocardial cells. A variety of methodologies have been assessed; delivery of purified stem cells, delivery of relatively unpurified bone marrow, systemic delivery of stem cells, delivery of stem cells into the coronary artery, or delivery into the myocardium at surgery.

The results and applicability of this technology await the results of ongoing clinical trials.

Trans-myocardial vascularisation

This is as yet an unproven experimental technique mainly used for end-stage ischaemia untreatable by conventional surgery. At open surgery, laser beams burn holes through the myocardium in the hope that some of these will develop into 'vascular' channels which could take oxygenated blood from the left ventricular cavity to the myocardium of the left ventricle.

It is subject to trial evaluation at present but cannot be recommended for treatment as yet.

Further Reading

1. McFate Smith W. Epidemiology of congestive heart failure. *Am J Cardiol* 1985; **55**: 3A-8A

2. Poole-Wilson PA. History, definition and classification of heart failure. In: Poole-Wilson PA, Colucci WS, Massie BM, Chatterjee K, Coats AJS, eds. Heart Failure; *Scientific principles and clinical practice*. London: Churchill Livingstone, 1997; 269-278

3. Coats AJS, Poole-Wilson PA. The syndrome of heart failure. In: Weatherall DJ, Ledingham JGG, Warrell DA, eds. *Oxford Textbook of Medicine*. Oxford: Oxford University Press, 1996; 2228-2238

4. Ho K. Epidemiology of CHF. *JACC* 1992; (in press)

5. Firth BG, Dunnmon PM. Left ventricular dilatation and failure post-myocardial infarction: pathophysiology and possible pharmacological interventions. *Cardiovasc Drug Therapy* 1990; **4**: 1363-1374

6. Braunwald E. ACE inhibitors - a cornerstone of the treatment of heart failure. *New Engl J Med* 1991; **325**: 351-353

7. Tan LB. Clinical and research implications of new concepts in the assessment of cardiac pumping performance in heart failure. *Cardiovasc Res* 1987; **21**: 615-622

8. Cohn J, Johnson GR, Shabetai R, et al. Ejection fraction, peak exercise oxygen consumption, cardiothoracic ratio, ventricular arrhythmias, and plasma norepinephrine as determinants of prognosis in heart failure. *Circulation* 1993; **87 (Suppl. VI)**: 5-13

9. Petrie MC, Hogg K, Caruana L, McMurray JJ. Poor concordance of commonly used echocardiographic measures of left ventricular diastolic function in patients with suspected heart failure but preserved systolic function: is there a reliable echocardiographic measure of diastolic dysfunction? *Heart* May 2004; **90(5)**: 511-7

10. Clark A, Coats A. The mechanisms underlying the increased ventilatory response to exercise in chronic stable heart failure. *Eur Heart J* 1992; **13**: 1698-1708

11. Clark AL, Coats AJS. Changes in lower limb skeletal muscle and mechanisms of fatigue in CHF. *BAM* 1995; **5**: 349-358

12. Coats AJS, Clark AL, Piepoli M, Volterrani M, Poole-Wilson PA. Symptoms and quality of life in heart failure; the muscle hypothesis. *Brit Heart J* 1994; **72 (Suppl)**: S36-S39

13. Wei CM, Aarhus LL, Miller VM, et al. The action of C-type natriuretic peptide in isolated canine arteries and veins. *Am. J. Physiol* 1993; **264**: H71-H73

14. Pacher R, Stanek B, Hülsmann M, Koller-Strametz J, Berger R, Schuller M, Hartter E, Ogris E, Frey B, Heinz G, Maurer G. Prognostic impact of big endothelin-1 plasma concentrations compared with invasive hemodynamic evaluation in severe heart failure. *J Am Coll Cardiol* 1996; **27**: 633-641

15. Anand I, McMurray J, Cohn JN, Konstam MA, Notter T, Quitzau K, Ruschitzka F, Luscher TF; EARTH investigators. Long-term effects of darusentan on left-ventricular remodelling and clinical outcomes in the EndothelinA Receptor Antagonist Trial in Heart Failure (EARTH): randomised, double-blind, placebo-controlled trial. *Lancet* 2004 Jul 24; **364**(9431): 347-54

16. Moore DP, Weston AR, Hughes JM, Oakley CM, Cleland JG. Effects of increased inspired oxygen concentrations on exercise performance in chronic heart failure. *Lancet* 1992; **339**: 850-853

17. Clark AL, Coats AJS. Usefulness of arterial blood gas estimations during exercise in patients with chronic heart failure. *Brit Heart J* 1994; **71**: 528-530

18. Chua TP, Lalloo UG, Worsdell MY, Kharitonov S, Chung KF, Coats AJS. Airway and cough responsiveness and exhaled nitric oxide in non-smoking patients with stable chronic heart failure. *Brit Heart J* 1996; **76**: 144-149

19. Chua TP, Clark AL, Amadi AA, Coats AJS. Relation between chemosensitivity and the ventilatory response to exercise in chronic heart failure. *J Am Coll Cardiol* 1996; **27**: 650-657

20. Chua TP, Harrington D, Ponikowski P, Webb-Peploe K, Poole-Wilson PA, Coats AJS. Effects of dihydrocodeine on chemosensitivity and exercise tolerance in patients with chronic heart failure. *J Am Coll Cardiol* 1997; **29**: 147-152

21. Harris S, LeMaitre JP, Mackenzie G, Fox KA, Denvir MA. A randomised study of home-based electrical stimulation of the legs and conventional bicycle exercise training for patients with chronic heart failure. *Eur Heart J* 2003; **24**: 871-8

22. Coats AJS, Adamopoulos S. Neurohormonal mechanisms and the role of angiotensin-converting enzyme (ACE) inhibitors in heart failure. *Cardiovasc Drug Therapy* 1994; **8**: 685-692

23. Squire IB, O'Brien RJ, Demme B, Davies JE, Ng LL. N-terminal pro-atrial natriuretic peptide (N-ANP) and N-terminal pro-B-type natriuretic peptide (N-BNP) in the prediction of death and heart failure in unselected patients following acute myocardial infarction. *Clin Sci* 2004; **107**: 309-16

24. Anand IS, Fisher LD, Chiang YT, Latini R, Masson S, Maggioni AP, Glazer RD, Tognoni G, Cohn JN; Val-HeFT Investigators. Changes in brain natriuretic peptide and norepinephrine over time and mortality and morbidity in the Valsartan Heart Failure Trial (Val-HeFT). *Circulation* 2003 Mar 11; **107(9)**: 1278-83

25. Nicholls MG, Lainchbury JG, Richards AM, Troughton RW, Yandle TG. Brain natriuretic peptide-guided therapy for heart failure. *Ann Med* 2001 Sep; **33(6)**: 422-7

26. Kawakami R, Saito Y, Kishimoto I, Harada M, Kuwahara K, Takahashi N, Nakagawa Y, Nakanishi M, Tanimoto K, Usami S, Yasuno S, Kinoshita H, Chusho H, Tamura N, Ogawa Y, Nakao K. Overexpression of brain natriuretic peptide facilitates neutrophil infiltration and cardiac matrix metalloproteinase-9 expression after acute myocardial infarction. *Circulation* 2004; **110**: 3306-12

27. Colucci WS, Elkayam U, Horton DP, et al. Intravenous nesiritide, a natriuretic peptide, in the treatment of decompensated congestive heart failure. *N Engl J Med* 2000; **343**: 246-253

28. Beta-Blocker Evaluation of Survival Trial Investigators. A trial of the beta-blocker bucindolol in patients with advanced chronic heart failure. *N Engl J Med* 2001; **344**: 1659-67

29. The Xamoterol in Severe Heart Failure Study Group. Xamoterol in severe heart failure. *Lancet* 1990 Jul 7; **336 (8706)**: 1-6

30. Packer M, Carver JR, Rodeheffer RJ, Ivanhoe RJ, DiBianco R, Zeldis SM, Hendrix GH, Bommer WJ, Elkayam U, Kukin ML, et al . Effect of oral milrinone on mortality in severe chronic heart failure. The PROMISE Study Research Group. *N Engl J Med* 1991; **325**: 1468-1475

31. Perry G, Brown E, Thornton R, Shiva T, Hubbard J, Reddy KR, Doherty JE,III, Cardello FP, Fast A, Radford MJ, Folger JS, Bhaskar G, Zoble RG, Sridharan V, Sridharan MR, Loungani RR, Gheorghiade M, Hsieh A, Tommaso C, Mansuri M, Guess MA, Akhtar S, Wagner S, Hagan K. The effect of digoxin on mortality and morbidity in patients with heart failure. *N Engl J Med* 1997; **336**: 525-533

32. Cohn JN, Archibald DG, Ziesche S, Franciosa JA, Harston WE, Tristani FE, Dunkman WB, Jacobs W, Francis GS, Flohr KH, Goldman S, Cobb FR, Shah PM, Saunders R, Fletcher RD, Loeb HS, Hughes VC, Baker B. Effect of vasodilator therapy on mortality in chronic congestive heart failure. *New Engl J Med* 1986; **314**: 1547-1552

33. Cohn JN, Johnson G, Ziesche S, Cobb F, Francis G, Tristani F, Smith R, Dunkman WB, Loeb H, Wong M, Bhat G, Goldman S, Fletcher RD, Doherty J, Hughes CV, Carson P, Cintron G, Shabetai R, Haakenson C. A comparison of enalapril with hydralazine-isosorbide dinitrate in the treatment of chronic congestive heart failure. *New Engl J Med* 1991; **325**: 303-310

34. Granger CB, McMurray JJ, Yusuf S, Held P, Michelson EL, Olofsson B, Ostergren J, Pfeffer MA, Swedberg K; CHARM Investigators and Committees. Effects of candesartan in patients with chronic heart failure and reduced left-ventricular systolic function intolerant to angiotensin-converting-enzyme inhibitors: the CHARM-Alternative trial. *Lancet* 2003; **362**: 772-6

35. Pfeffer MA, McMurray JJ, Velazquez EJ, Rouleau JL, Kober L, Maggioni AP, Solomon SD, Swedberg K, Van de Werf F, White H, Leimberger JD, Henis M, Edwards S, Zelenkofske S, Sellers MA, Califf RM; Valsartan in Acute Myocardial Infarction Trial Investigators. Valsartan, captopril, or both in myocardial infarction complicated by heart failure, left ventricular dysfunction, or both. *N Engl J Med* 2003; **349**: 1893-906

36. Anand I, McMurray JJV, Whitmore J, et al. Anaemia and its Relationship to Clinical Outcome in Heart Failure. *Circulation* 2004; **110**: 149-153

37. Silverberg DS, Wexler D, Blum M, et al. The effect of correction of anaemia in diabetics and non-diabetics with severe resistant congestive heart failure and chronic renal failure by subcutaneous erythropoietin and intravenous iron. *Nephrol Dial Transplant* 2003; **18**: 141-46

38. Sullivan MJ, Higginbotham MB, Cobb FR. Exercise training in patients with chronic heart failure delays ventilatory anaerobic threshold and improves submaximal exercise performance. *Circulation* 1989; **79**: 324-329

39. Sullivan MJ, Higginbotham MB, Cobb FR. Exercise training in patients with severe left ventricular dysfunction: Hemodynamic and metabolic effects. *Circulation* 1988; **78**: 506-515

40. Coats AJS, Adamopoulos S, Meyer TE, Conway J, Sleight P. Effects of physical training in chronic heart failure. *Lancet* 1990; **335**: 63-66

41. Coats AJS. The "Muscle Hypothesis" of Chronic Heart Failure. *J. Molecular and Cellular Cardiology* 1996; **28**: 2255-2262

42. Packer M, Bristow MR, Cohn JN, Colucci WS, Fowler MB, Gilbert EM, Shusterman NH. The effect of carvedilol on morbidity and mortality in patients with chronic heart failure. *N Engl J Med* 1996; **334**: 1349-1355

43. MacMahon S, Sharpe N, Doughty R, Krum H, Tonkin A, Trotter A, Burton R, Garrett J, Lane G, Owensby D, Ryan J, Shepherd J, Singh B, Jackson B, Rudge

G, Stephensen J, Woodhouse S, Davidson P, Turner J, Walsh W, Bradbury J, Hamer A, Cross D, Hall C. Randomised, placebo-controlled trial of carvedilol in patients with congestive heart failure due to ischaemic heart disease. *Lancet* 1997; **349**: 375-380

44. The Cardiac Insufficiency Bisoprolol Study II (CIBIS-II): a randomised trial. *Lancet* 1999; **353**: 9-13

45. Hjalmarson A, Goldstein S, Fagerberg B, Wedel H, Waagstein F, Kjekshus J, Wikstrand J, El Allaf D, Vitovec J, Aldershvile J, Halinen M, Dietz R, Neuhaus KL, Janosi A, Thorgeirsson G, Dunselman PH, Gullestad L, Kuch J, Herlitz J, Rickenbacher P, Ball S, Gottlieb S, Deedwania P. Effects of controlled-release metoprolol on total mortality, hospitalisations, and well-being in patients with heart failure: the Metoprolol CR/XL Randomized Intervention Trial in congestive heart failure (MERIT-HF). MERIT-HF Study Group. *JAMA* 2000; **283**: 1295-302

46. Flather MD, Shibata MC, Coats AJ, Van Veldhuisen DJ, Parkhomenko A, Borbola J, Cohen-Solal A, Dumitrascu D, Ferrari R, Lechat P, Soler-Soler J, Tavazzi L, Spinarova L, Toman J, Bohm M, Anker SD, Thompson SG, Poole-Wilson PA; SENIORS Investigators. Randomized trial to determine the effect of nebivolol on mortality and cardiovascular hospital admission in elderly patients with heart failure (SENIORS). *Eur Heart J* 2005; **26**: 215-25

47. Pitt B, Zannad F, Remme WJ et al for the Randomized Aldactone Evaluation Study Investigators. The effect of spironolactone on morbidity and mortality in patients with severe heart failure. *N Engl J Med* 1999; **341**: 709-717

48. Pitt B, Remme W, Zannad F et al. Eplerenone, a selective aldosterone blocker, in patients with left ventricular dysfunction after myocardial infarction. *N Engl J Med* 2003; **348**: 1309-1321

49. Julian DG, Camm AJ, Frangin G, Janse MJ, Munoz A, Schwartz PJ, Simon P. Randomised trial of effect of amiodarone on mortality in patients with left-ventricular dysfunction after recent myocardial infarction: EMIAT. *Lancet* 1997; **349**: 667-674

50. Cairns JA, Connolly SJ, Roberts R, Gent M. Randomised trial of outcome after myocardial infarction in patients with frequent or repetitive ventricular premature depolarisations: CAMIAT. *Lancet* 1997; **349**: 675-682

51. Bardy GH, Lee KL, Mark DB, Poole JE, Packer DL, Boineau R, Domanski M, Troutman C, Anderson J, Johnson G, McNulty SE, Clapp-Channing N, Davidson-Ray LD, Fraulo ES, Fishbein DP, Luceri RM, Ip JH; Sudden Cardiac Death in Heart Failure Trial (SCD-HeFT) Investigators. Amiodarone or an implantable cardioverter-defibrillator for congestive heart failure. *N Engl J Med* 2005; **352**: 225-37

52. Feldman AM, Bristow MR, Parmley WW, Carson PE, Pepine CJ, Gilbert EM, Strobeck JE, Hendrix GH, Powers ER, Bain RB, White BG, for the Vesnarinone Study Group. Effects of vesnarinone on morbidity and mortality in patients with heart failure. *New Engl J Med* 1993; **329**: 149-155

53. Cleland JG, Poole-Wilson P. Is aspirin safe in heart failure? More data. *Heart* 1996 Apr; **75(4)**: 426

54. The CONSENSUS Trial Study Group. Effects of enalapril on mortality in severe congestive heart failure: results of the Cooperative North Scandinavian Enalapril Survival Study. *New Engl J Med* 1987; **316**: 1429-1435

55. The SOLVD Investigators. Effect of enalapril on survival in patients with reduced left ventricular ejection fractions and congestive heart failure. *New Engl J Med* 1991; **325**: 293-302

56. The SOLVD Investigators. Effect of enalapril on mortality and the development of heart failure in asymptomatic patients with reduced left ventricular ejection fractions. *New Engl J Med* 1992; **327**: 685-691

57. Swedberg K, Held P, Kjekshus J, Rasmussen K, Rydén L, Wedel H, on behalf of the CONSENSUS II study group. Effects of the early administration of enalapril on mortality in patients with acute myocardial infarction. Results of the Cooperative New Scandinavian Enalapril Survival Study II (CONSENSUS II). *New Engl J Med* 1992; **327**: 678-684

58. Pfeffer MA, Braunwald E, Moyé LA, Basta L, Brown EJ, Jr., Cuddy TE, Davis BR, Geltman EM, Goldman S, Flaker GC, Klein M, Lamas GA, Packer M, Rouleau J, Rouleau JL, Rutherford J, Wertheimer JH, Hawkins CM, on behalf of the SAVE investigators. Effect of captopril on mortality and morbidity in patients with left ventricular dysfunction after myocardial infarction. Results of the Survival and Ventricular Enlargement Trial. *New Engl J Med* 1992; **327**: 669-677

59. The Acute Infarction Ramipril Efficacy (AIRE) Study Investigators. Effect of ramipril on mortality and morbidity of survivors of acute myocardial infarction with clinical evidence of heart failure. *Lancet* 1993; **342**: 821-828

60. Gruppo Italiano per lo Studio della Sopravvivenza nell'Infarto Micardio. GISSI-3: effects of lisinopril and transdermal glyceryl trinitrate singly and together on 6-week mortality and ventricular function after acute myocardial infarction. *Lancet* 1994; **343**: 1115-1122

61. SIS-4 Collaborative Group. ISIS-4: A randomised factorial trial assessing early oral captopril, oral mononitrate, and intravenous magnesium sulphate in 58050 patients with suspected acute myocardial infarction. *Lancet* 1995; **345**: 669-685

62. Dickstein K, Kjekshus J. Comparison of the Effects of Losartan and Captopril on Mortality and Morbidity in patients following Acute Myocardial Infarction: The OPTIMAAL Trial. *Lancet* 2002; **360**: 752-60

63. McMurray JJV, Ostergren J, Swedberg K, et al. Effects of candesartan in patients with CHF and reduced left ventricular systolic function taking angiotensin converting enzyme inhibitors – the CHARM Added trial. *Lancet* 2003; **362**: 767-771

64. Yusuf S, Pfeffer MA, Swedberg K, et al. Effects of candesartan in patients with chronic heart failure and preserved left ventricular ejection fraction – the CHARM preserved trial. *Lancet* 2003; **362**: 777-781

65. National Institute for Clinical Excellence. Management of chronic heart failure in adults in primary and secondary care. Clinical guideline 5 (2003)

66. MacFadyen RJ, Lees KR, Reid JL. Differences in first dose response to angiotensin converting enzyme inhibition in congestive heart failure: a placebo controlled study. *Brit Heart J* 1991; **66**: 206-211

67. Squire IB, RJ MacFadyen, JL Reid, A Devlin, KR Lees. Differing early blood pressure and renin angiotensin system responses to the first dose of Angiotensin Converting Enzyme inhibitors in congestive heart failure. *J Cardiovasc Pharmacol* 1996; **27**: 657-666

Index